The Energetics of Voice Dialogue

The Energetics of Voice Dialogue

*An In-Depth Exploration of the
Energetic Aspects of
Transformational Psychology*

ROBERT STAMBOLIEV

LifeRhythm

Library of Congress Cataloging-in-Publication Data

Stamboliev, Robert.
The energetics of voice dialogue: an in-depth exploration of the energetic
aspects of transformational psychology / Robert Stamboliev.

Originally presented as the author's thesis (M.A.)--William Lyon University,
1988.
Includes bibliographical references.
ISBN 0-940795-12-4 : S10.95
1. Archetype (Psychology) 2. Self-talk. 3. Role playing. 4. Voice dialogue.
   5. Transformational psychology. I. Title.
[BF 175.5.A72S73 1992]
158'.9--dc20   92-1112
                                                          CIP

Copyright © 1992
LIFERHYTHM
P.O. Box 806
Mendocino CA 95460
707/937-1825 Fax: 707/937-3052

ACKNOWLEDGEMENTS

I wish to express my deep appreciation for the inspiration received from Drs. Hal and Sidra Stone and for the continued assistance and support of Dr. Hilary Anderson.

I wish to thank Dr. Jerien Koolbergen and Dr. Berenda Dekkers for their continuing support in the Netherlands and Wentzle Ruml, III, for his editorial assistance.

In particular, I want to thank my mother, Wil Petroff-van Gurp, for her unwavering support and understanding throughout my entire study.

And, finally, I wish to acknowledge all the clients and workshop participants with whom I have worked over the last few years. Without them this study would not have been possible.

Robert Stamboliev

TABLE OF CONTENTS

INTRODUCTION TO THE ENERGETICS OF VOICE DIALOGUE

We are very pleased to write an introduction to Robert Stamboliev's book, *The Energetics of Voice Dialogue.* We have long been familiar with his personal work and with his remarkable ability as a teacher and trainer. In this book, he also establishes himself as a writer. Building upon his extensive background in Tai Chi, Robert has combined his knowledge of energetics together with his understanding and experience with the Voice Dialogue process and the theory of selves. The result is a book that will be invaluable to anyone interested in the study of selves and the Voice Dialogue process in particular.

Robert attended our very first Voice Dialogue workshop in Den Haag in the fall of 1982. Hal gave a lecture at the Kosmos, a growth center in Amsterdam, on Voice Dialogue. Robert had studied the use of the voice and sound for many years and he came to Hal's lecture quite accidentally, if, in fact, there is such a thing as an accident. Following the lecture, he signed up for the workshop and thus it was that he began his own training and a new phase in his own personal journey.

Since that time, Voice Dialogue has become a worldwide movement and Holland has been a major center for the transmission of the work. We have taken great pains to not let it solidify into a hard form, the fate of many approaches to growth and personal transformation. It is for this reason that we have taken the strong position that there be no certification of Voice Dialogue therapists.

It is impossible to separate Voice Dialogue from the dream process, from interpersonal dynamics, from symbolic visualization, and most importantly, from the knowledge and experience of energetics. It is not a system unto itself. As a method, and as a philosophical approach to consciousness, it can be integrated into any system of work, both methodologically and theoretically. This is exactly what is happening around the world today. Robert has developed his own unique style of facilitation, teaching and training and the core of his work stems from his experience and knowledge of the energetic process.

When one first learns the Voice Dialogue process, it appears to be a form, a technique like many other techniques. What one soon discovers is that the selves that we are reaching for are energetic realities. They are literally vibrating systems and it is the task of the Voice Dialogue facilitator to learn to recognize and resonate with them. This is the heart of the work. The Voice Dialogue facilitator is essentially an energy dancer, sometimes active, sometimes quiet, sometimes yang and sometimes yin. Not only is the facilitator an energy dancer, he or she has also learned to induct energies that live in the unconscious and bring them to the surface when that is appropriate. The trained facilitator can induct these energies in the subject by simply tuning in to his or her internal energy system, and allowing it to be present until the corresponding energy emerges in the subject.

Thus the trained facilitator can teach the subject to dance the many dances of the different selves of the subject whose job it is to protect each of us as we journey through life. To take it yet a step deeper, the trained facilitator ultimately realizes that all energy is God, and that the dance of the many selves is, in truth, the dance of the many gods and goddesses who inhabit our being.

Robert has become an energy dancer, and it is this sensitivity to energy that he has mastered and that he describes so well in this book. In a very practical way, he shows how the knowledge of, and sensitivity to, the energetic process can be used quite directly in the practice of Voice Dialogue. He describes quite systematically, the steps taken by the facilitator in preparing for and carrying out the work. In short, it is a book well written and well worth your time to read. We are pleased to have played some part in Robert's journey.

Hal Stone, Ph.D. and Sidra Stone, Ph.D.
Thera—Albion, California, November, 1991

1

ABOUT VOICE DIALOGUE

I n one of those seemingly fated moments of my life, I walked into a well-
known growth center in Amsterdam in December 1982, to attend a lecture on Voice Dialogue by Hal Stone, Ph. D. I had been working as a
voice coach for some time, and I expected to hear him talk about working
with the human voice.

Instead, Dr. Stone was talking about Transformational Psychology and
a method, which he called Voice Dialogue, that deals with the "inner" voices
rather than the "outer" voice. Despite my expectations, I was very interested by his talk and was fascinated by the demonstration he performed, with
a woman from the audience as his subject.

In the next two days, I participated in the introductory workshop in
Voice Dialogue led by Hal Stone, Ph.D. and Sidra Winkelman, Ph.D.,* his
wife and colleague. Together, they had originally developed the method
as a means of communicating better with one another.

Voice Dialogue is a synthesis of many other approaches towards the
transformation of consciousness. I had studied the work of Krishnamurti. I
had practised T'ai Chi Ch'uan and Indian music for a number of years, had
completed a two-year Gestalt-therapy training, and was at that time also
involved with a theatre group that emphasized the use of the human voice.
Although I had a sense that these various disciplines were somehow related to one another, I found it difficult to bring them together in a satisfying
perspective. I discovered very quickly, however, that the Transformational

*Now Sidra Stone, Ph.D.

Psychology introduced by Stone and Winkelman gave me that perspective. Through Voice Dialogue, I was able to integrate my various experiences with different traditions.

Happily for me, Voice Dialogue also proved to be a good tool that allowed me to put to practical use, in working with its inclusive method, all the skills I had developed through the practice of these disciplines.

The inclusive quality of the method is due to two facts: that the different "voices" in Voice Dialogue are viewed as having the fundamental common denominator of all being energy patterns, and that working with them demands a particular "energetic" approach. I also found that, in order to objectify the different energy patterns in the subject, the Voice Dialogue facilitator really engages energetically with the subject by tuning in and resonating with his own corresponding energy patterns.

In October 1983, I went to Los Angeles to study Transformational Psychology with Stone and Winkelman at the Academy of Delos. I studied with them for eight months, taking part in all their groups and seminars on Voice Dialogue, dreamwork, energetics, and visualization. Subsequently, in 1984, I returned to the Netherlands to teach what I had learned.

By 1988, I had trained many people, a number of whom are now leading their own Voice Dialogue groups. What I have observed in training these people, is that those who are what Dr. Stone calls "energy sensitives" pick up the techniques quite naturally, while others need training specifically designed to develop the energetic aspect of the work.

Stone and Winkelman have published a Voice Dialogue manual entitled *Embracing Our Selves,* in which they develop the theoretical framework of the method and give guidelines for the facilitation process. In addition, there have been a number of academic studies developed that discuss the Stone-Winkelman consciousness model and the interplay of subpersonality work. They have more recently published *Embracing Each Other* and Dr. Stone has written *Embracing Heaven and Earth, A Personal Odyssey.*

Although Drs. Stone and Winkelman include energetic training in their seminars, they have not elaborated a great deal on this aspect of the work in their book, nor have the other studies centered on this aspect. Because the energetic aspect is such an essential element of the method, I feel that its development needs more attention.

When the facilitator does not have enough proficiency in the use of energetics, the work may have a great deal of mental content, but the emotional-physical base of the energy patterns involved in the sessions will not be sufficiently tapped to bring about solid and lasting transformational changes.

In my Voice Dialogue training groups in the Netherlands, I have found that personal induction by an experienced facilitator at a sufficiently deep level of consciousness is necessary, in order that a "core of energy" can be touched and dialogued, and, therefore, acknowledged and utilized for transformation. Furthermore, I have come to the conclusion that specific energetic training—based on T'ai Chi Ch'uan and the esoteric tradition that works with body energy fields and the energy centers (chakras)—greatly help people to become aware of the energetics of Voice Dialogue.

For the understanding of the T'ai Chi principles that seem to match this transformational work so well, I owe a great deal to the various T'ai Chi teachers I have had, especially Dr. Kwee Swan Ho, of Amsterdam, and Master Benjamin P.J. Lo, of San Francisco.

In this study, I hope, first of all, to clarify the energetics of Voice Dialogue, and, in addition, to present perspectives from T'ai Chi Ch'uan and esoteric traditions that will aid the practitioner of Voice Dialogue to develop a deeper energetic sensitivity for the method.

DIFFERENT VIEWS ON "TRANSFORMATION"

Although a good many teachers, therapists, and scholars such as C.G. Jung, Abraham Maslow and Jiddu Krishnamurti have developed perspectives on the transformation of consciousness, they perceived this transformation as an essentially individual work, to be carried out through the agency of personal crises, prolonged meditation and contemplation. They stressed the idea that, beyond a certain point, individuals must strive on their own rather than pursue continued dialogue with a teacher or therapist. In this connection, it is interesting to note that Maslow quoted Carl Rogers as reporting that successful therapy raises the average score of a patient on the Willoughby Maturity Scale from the 25th to the 50th percentile. Maslow then asks himself, "Who has to raise him to the 75th or the 100th percentile? Are there new principles or techniques necessary?"

Since 1950, there have been several different schools that focus on various aspects of our human nature, often to the exclusion of other aspects.

Within these different schools, there are methods that focus on the physical body and our emotions, such as Gestalt therapy and Bioenergetics. There are methods that work with the imagination and creative arts, such as established Jungian psychological techniques, as well as those of Psychosynthesis, stressing transpersonal dimensions of consciousness. There are other disciplines, such as those developed by Gurdjieff and Ouspensky, that lay stress on a variety of techniques to explore the various centers of consciousness. Perhaps the most inclusive approach that can give us a full view and experience of the totality of our being is the recently developed tool called Voice Dialogue. This approach is a synthesis of Humanistic Psychology and Transpersonal Psychology and includes an energy component, called Energetics, that distinguishes it truly as a Transformational Psychology.

ENERGETICS

Most of the written materials on the Voice Dialogue technique have developed along the lines of discussion of the consciousness model and the interplay of subpersonality work. Therefore, the purpose of this study is to clarify the energetic nature of Voice Dialogue and the importance of the energetics aspect in the transformation of energy patterns in psychological work. An additional purpose is to incorporate selected materials drawn from the traditions of T'ai Chi Ch'uan and the esoteric healing systems that can aid the Voice Dialogue facilitator to work more energetically with the method. It is expected that this approach will gain theoretical and practical application in the larger work of Transformational Psychology.

REVIEW OF THE LITERATURE

In developing the theme of this thesis, particular works have been especially valuable. In the first place, the Stone-Winkelman book, *Embracing Our Selves* was the most important source for their ideas about consciousness and transformation, as well as describing the method of Voice Dialogue itself. Also of great importance were the notes collected from the seminars with Drs. Stone and Winkelman that I have attended over the years.

The psychology of Carl Gustav Jung provides probably the most basic perspective for the theoretical framework of Voice Dialogue, and the key points in Jungian psychology revolve around the concept of individuation. The process of individuation is developed through reconciling different and sometimes opposing trends within the psyche. These trends come from the postulation that, within every human being, there exist both masculine and feminine characteristics, known as the Animus and the Anima. The Jungian tradition also postulates that there are four basic personality types—the thinking type, the feeling (subjective) type, the sensation (practical) type, and the intuitive type—and that we identify with different types as compensatory functions to adapt to our life circumstances. This adaptation is referred to as our Persona, and it manifests either with an introverted attitude—that is, oriented toward the subjective, inner reality—or an extraverted attitude—oriented toward the external, objective reality. The rest of the functions, as well as the male or female portion of the psyche, are relegated to balance out a person's outward attitude. The unconscious produces dreams and fantasies that emphasize the opposite demands.

Beyond this area, there is the collective unconscious, wherein lie the substantial images and ideas that are common to all people, shared by the entire human race. These primordial possibilities for action, or psychic predispositions for the shaping of response, are known as Archetypes. They give rise to the symbols that the unconscious uses in its depiction of the material within it, and our associations with what we experience as the outer reality. Thus, associative techniques—such as Jung's early work with word associations, active imagination, dreams, and the use of art—which are ultimately symbolic in nature, become important in reaching into the unconscious and helping to bring about a harmony with the Ego, the conscious part of the personality.

Part of this process also involves coming to terms with what Jung called the Shadow—described as the unacceptable, repressed, undesirable tendencies within us, which we prefer not to recognize. These tendencies, repressed in the unconscious, usually become projected onto other people. It is through the examination of this behavior, and the process of individuation, that a harmony with, and an expression of, the self is achieved.

Specific references utilized for background in Jungian ideas and concepts were two books by C.G. Jung himself, *Modern Man in Search of a Soul* and *Memories, Dreams, Reflections*; Christopher Monte's *Beneath the Mask*; and Frieda Fordham's *An Introduction to Jung's Psychology*.

The concept of Awareness is utilized by most eastern and western spiritual traditions. In this century, it was Jiddu Krishnamurti who stressed the importance of the awareness level and who had a strong impact on my overall understanding. His concept of "choiceless awareness" is particularly relevant to the Voice Dialogue process. He claimed that there is no mystic way that can be taught. Having a total awareness of the moment, outside the boundaries of time, is what matters. The fundamental theme of Krishnamurti's works repeats consistently: "There is hope in man, not in society, not in systems, organized religious systems, but in you and me." His main way of reaching the stage of freedom is to practice "choiceless awareness."

The liberating process must begin with the choiceless awareness of what you will and of your reactions to the symbol system which tells you

*that you ought or ought not, to will it. Through this choiceless aware-
ness, as it penetrates the successive layers of the Ego and its associated
subconscious, will come love and understanding, but of another order
than that with which we are ordinarily familiar. This choiceless awareness—at every moment and in all circumstances of life—is the only effective meditation (Krishnamurti, 1954, p. 222)*

What stands out in Krishnamurti's perspective, is the intensity of focusing
on the question, whether the mind can free itself from its self-created bond-
age, and whether this can bring about a breakthrough into another level
of Awareness.

*All other questions are irrelevant and prevent the mind from attend-
ing to that one question. There is no attention when there is a motive,
the pressure to achieve, to realize; that is, when the mind is seeking a
result, an end. The mind will discover the solution of this problem, not
through arguments, opinions, convictions or beliefs, but through the very
intensity of the question itself. (Krishnamurti, 1968, p. 285)*

The system for self-realization of G.I. Gurdjieff and P.D. Ouspensky is
also based on the premise that we are made up out of parts. Without an
awareness of these parts, change and transformation are considered impossible. In *Psychological Commentaries on the Teaching of Gurdjieff and
Ouspensky*, Maurice Nicoll, who was a student of both, notes the following:

*When a man begins to observe himself from the angle that he is not
one but many, he begins the work on his being. He cannot do this if he
remains under the conviction that he is one, for then he will not be able
to separate himself from himself, for he will take everything in him, every thought, mood, feeling, impulse, desire, emotion, and so on, as himself—that is, as "I." But if he begins to observe himself, he will then, at
that moment, become two—an observing side and an observed
side...Unless he...struggles to make this division more and more distinct,
he will never be able to shift from where he is...—the crowd of separate
"I"s...both useful and useless—will have...equal rights and be equally
protected by him because he will be quite unable to distinguish them from
one another since he takes them all as himself. (Nicoll, 1952, p. 21-22)*

In this context, the "observer" and that which is being observed, are analogous to the Stone and Winkelman's Awareness level and the many different energy patterns or subpersonalities.

For developing the ideas and practice of energetics in relation to Voice Dialogue, I have been greatly influenced by the eastern and western esoteric traditions. From the vast literature on the subject, I have particularly focused on the work of the late W.E. Butler, *How to Read the Aura*, to describe the basic assumptions of these traditions regarding our body energy fields.

W.E. Butler was a well known clairvoyant and the leader of an esoteric school in England. In the above publication, he describes the structure of the aura, with its various energy centers, called chakras (the Sanskrit term for wheels). The book is clearly written, based on a lifelong experience as a psychic and healer.

Valuable notes, gathered from practical training in energetics I received from Hal Stone and from Carolyn Conger, Ph.D., a psychologist, psychic and healer, form an important collection of data for this work. The energy work used by Hal Stone and Carolyn Conger is closely connected to that of W. Brugh Joy, M.D., who gives a personal description of his work, in his book, *Joy's Way: A Map for the Transformational Journey*. This publication not only describes energy work but also is a report of Brugh Joy's personal odyssey. He describes his own transformation from an orthodox physician to an unorthodox spiritual and psychic healer. Brugh Joy draws conclusions about the transformational process based on his own experiences, as well as the experiences of hundreds who attended his conferences. His writings on the subject have served as an inspiration to many other therapists. He also seems to be the first person to have used the term "Transformational Psychology." In personal correspondence with Linda A. Nifenger he wrote:

...The term Transformational Psychology was coined in 1975 when I was attempting to describe my exploration of therapeutic psychology/psychiatry which reflected integration of spiritual as well as physical, emotional and mental aspects of health and disease. Access to expanded states of awareness was the major criterion which differentiated Transformational Psychology from other more conventional modes of approach. I have no idea if the term was previously used by others. (Nifenger, 1985, p. 35)

In *Joy's Way*, Brugh Joy offers specific exercises and techniques which may be employed in a therapy session by a transformational psychologist. In exploring how the principles of T'ai Chi Ch'uan relate to Transformational Psychology, I draw on my experience in practicing T'ai Chi Ch'uan with different masters. The only literature on the subject that the masters consider important is known simply as the T'ai Chi Ch'uan Classics, a collection of writings spanning almost one thousand years. The T'ai Chi Ch'uan Classics were translated into English in 1979 by the well-known T'ai Chi Ch'uan master Benjamin Pang Jeng Lo, together with his students, Martin Inn, Robert Amacker and Susan Foe, and were published as *The Essence of T'ai Chi Ch'uan*. I have used this translation of the T'ai Chi Ch'uan Classics to clarify and highlight the different principles that I will describe in Chapter 3. Because of its lofty goals and profound insights, the T'ai Chi Ch'uan Classics is considered a book of wisdom.

> *In the Orient, if a book which addresses itself to philosophical questions has merit, later scholars add their own commentaries. Over the centuries, as commentary is added to commentary, they come to be accepted as part of the work itself. New ideas are added and old ones are dropped as the text comes under the scrutiny of each succeeding generation. This organic process of addition and deletion tends to glean out the ideas found to be the wisest and most useful so that each proverb is like a telegram from past T'ai Chi Ch'uan practitioners. (Lo, et al., 1979, p. 8)*

One of the major goals of Taoism is health and longevity—"to live forever and be forever young." To achieve this purpose, one must follow the Tao (way or path), which means harmonizing with nature and the universe. This harmonization must be both external and internal. T'ai Chi Ch'uan is a method by which external affairs are regulated (self-defense) while the chi (vital energy) is cultivated. The Classics refer to both of these ideas. Yet, since the framework of T'ai Chi Ch'uan is that of the martial arts, everything in T'ai Chi Ch'uan must stand up to the most rigorous martial analysis. The T'ai Chi Ch'uan Classics are an attempt to state the irrevocable principles of Taoism in terms of martial arts.

2

THE CONSCIOUSNESS MODEL

I n this chapter, a brief historical overview will be given of the development of certain perspectives that led to the new Transformational Psychology and the consciousness model of Stone and Winkelman.

HISTORICAL PERSPECTIVE

In the 1960's, the so-called "Third Force" in psychology emerged alongside classical psychoanalysis and behaviorism. Mainly through the work of Abraham Maslow, this Third Force became known as Humanistic Psychology.

In Humanistic Psychology, consciousness, after having been a taboo for years, became the subject of study in which the re-establishment of the unity of body and mind was the most important emphasis. In this way, many therapies emerged that were aimed at experiencing body energies. In them, it was important to get a so-called "grounding" and, therefore, to center on the experience–we are living on the earth and the earth energies are within us.

Although this "Third Force" was also aimed at growth and self-actualization, Maslow himself was pessimistic about the outcome of using therapy alone for the process. He said: "You can go into therapy, or participate in growth oriented groups, but you will reach a point where you have to do it all by yourself." Beyond this point, he saw meditation as the only method for reaching higher states. After having come to these conclusions, he also became a co-creator with others in the founding of Transpersonal Psychology in the 70's.

The school of Transpersonal Psychology developed its own conscious-ness model, which was influenced by concepts from the exact sciences as well as eastern traditions. Consciousness was now viewed as a dynamic energy system. In this model, consciousness is seen as having different layers, so that there are various levels of consciousness that one may experience. The transcendental, spiritual experience was also seen as a level of consciousness. Under the influence of eastern spiritual traditions, such as Yoga, Sufism, and Buddhism, the idea of consciousness as energy was well developed. Much attention was also directed to dreams, hypnosis and altered states of consciousness, with data based on psychedelic experience, visualization, and meditation.

In addition, the theory of the brain's division into left and right hemispheres developed. In this theory, the left hemisphere was seen as governing linear thinking and time, while the right hemisphere had the function of intuition and imagination. Within the last ten years, however, a new perspective, which has been called Transformational Psychology, has emerged. This perspective can be seen as a synthesis of the previous approaches, integrating both body, emotion and spiritual energies with the foundation of energetics as a potent agent for transformation of consciousness.

Important exponents of this new Transformational Psychology are Hal Stone, Ph.D., and Sidra Winkelman, Ph.D. In his autobiography, *Embracing Heaven and Earth*, Stone describes his journey from being a Jungian analyst to being a Transformational Psychologist. Both Stone and Winkelman in their respective ways were involved in the above-mentioned development of growth and "grounding" therapies in the 1960's (Gestalt therapy and neo-Reichian work) and healing and energy work in the seventies, where unconditional love was the key idea. Later, they also disengaged from this last approach and began looking for a synthesis. They started Delos, a psychological corporation, in Los Angeles, where Stone led the trainings and Winkelman was director of their clinic. In 1986, they moved to Albion, California, and they now dedicate their time to writing and to extended teaching engagements in various training centers around the world that have been inspired by their work. They teach their consciousness model and the method they developed, called Voice Dialogue. Work with dreams, visualizations and body energy fields is incorporated into the larger perspective of the consciousness model.

DEFINITION OF CONSCIOUSNESS

In this consciousness model, consciousness is understood as both the awareness and the experience of energy patterns.

When Stone and Winkelman speak about consciousness they are implying a consciousness process. In this regard, they state:

What we will be defining...is not consciousness but the consciousness process. We will be calling it consciousness, but we are not talking about a condition of being. As far as we are concerned, one does not become simply conscious: consciousness is not simply something that we strive to achieve. Consciousness is a process that we must live out—an evolutionary process continually changing, fluctuating, from one moment to the next. (Stone and Winkelman, 1985, p. 17)

The consciousness process evolves on three distinct levels. One level is that of Awareness. The second level is that of the experience of the different parts, called Subpersonalities or Energy Patterns. The third level is the level of the Ego.

Stone and Winkelman define the Awareness level as "the capacity of witnessing life in all its aspects without evaluating or judging the energy patterns being witnessed and without having the need to control the outcome of an event."

The second level of the consciousness process is the experience of energy patterns. In this perspective, everything in life is seen as an energy pattern of one kind or another. "These particular energy patterns relate to our own internal states, be they physical, emotional, mental or spiritual. The energy patterns may vary from a vague feeling, or a barely discernible sensation, to a fully developed part or sub-personality." In defining energy patterns, Stone and Winkelman say that: "The term 'energy pattern' encompasses parts that are personally conditioned (sub-personalities) as well as parts that are based on a genetic predisposition (archetypes)."

The third level of the consciousness process is the Ego. Stone and Winkelman use the traditional definition of the Ego as the executive function of the psyche, or choice-maker.

Ideally, the Ego would receive its information both from the Awareness level and from the experience of the different energy patterns. What Stone and Winkelman discovered in their work, is that very few people can make real choices. In their terms:

The Ego has succumbed to a combination of different subpersonalities which have taken over its executive function. Thus, what, in fact, is functioning as the Ego, may be a combination of what has been referred to as one's Protector/Controller, Pusher, Pleaser, Perfectionist and Inner Critic. Therefore, we say that the Ego is identified *with these particular patterns. (Stone and Winkelman, 1985, p. 21)*

Stone and Winkelman see the consciousness process as one of crucial importance for individuals to become "aware" of the energy patterns their Ego is identified with. This leads to a refinement of the Ego. This concept of the "Aware Ego," which Stone and Winkelman introduced, is definitely an innovation. In their words, "As one moves forward in the consciousness process, the Ego becomes a more Aware Ego. As a more Aware Ego, it is in a better position to make real choices." Therefore, in this consciousness model, the three levels described are interlinked closely.

Consciousness Model

The model itself is best conceptualized by thinking about consciousness as an ongoing flow of psychic energy through the life process. Stone and Winkelman use the old model of the Lemniscate to show this flow of energies.

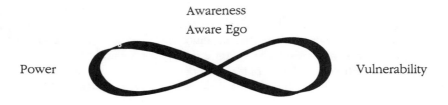

Awareness
Aware Ego

Power   Vulnerability

The energy flows between the two poles, which we may call minus and plus, Yin and Yang, vulnerability and power.

According to Stone and Winkelman, this process is archetypal and is part of the human condition. At the Yin pole, belong subpersonalities like the Vulnerable Child, Rebellious Son or Daughter, whereas, at the Yang pole belong power subpersonalities like the Father, Mother, Controller. Stone and Winkelman use this model especially to demonstrate the bonding patterns and energy flow that happen in relationships. In relationships, the Yin pole of one partner relates and responds to the Yang pole of the other partner, and vice versa.

This archetypal bonding happens in all relationships, be they man-woman, man-man, or woman-woman, and as an archetypal process it can be experienced as comfortable or as restrictive.

As can be observed, there is continuous flow between opposite energies. The Awareness level does not contain these mathematics; it can be aware of what is going on, but it is seen as being of a fundamentally different nature. The Aware Ego has access both to the experience of energy patterns and to the awareness level itself, as well as being able to communicate with other persons outside of the energetic bonding patterns. For example, a person who has developed an Aware Ego can experience his own energy patterns, as well as experiencing other people's energy patterns, while maintaining his own awareness.

AIMS OF TRANSFORMATIONAL PSYCHOLOGY

Clearly, the aim of Transformational Psychology is a transformation—a change in composition and character—of consciousness. According to Stone and Winkelman, intentional transformation can happen on the three levels of consciousness: Awareness, Experience of Energy Patterns, and the Ego.

I: Awareness

At the level of Awareness, one witnesses as in a detached perspective, more aspects of the self and its environment than before intentional consciousness work began. One becomes aware of Energies that the Ego was identified with, and of Energies that have been repressed. One can also develop more awareness of the body and the energy fields.

II: Experience of Energy Patterns

On the level of the Experience of Energy Patterns, several different changes may occur. Energies with which we have been *identified*, that have become stronger and larger, completely running our lives (Stone and Winkelman refer to them as the "Primary Selves"), can give up some control, begin to lose their dictatorial quality and be satisfied with a more constructive task. For example, an Inner Critic that has been beating us up ninety percent of the time, criticizing us on everything we do, can change through transformational work and become part of the analytical mind.

Energies that have been repressed for a long time, being pushed into the unconscious, are referred to as *disowned selves*. The concept of disowned selves was originated by psychologist Nathaniel Brandon, who was particularly interested in the disowning of emotionality and passion in our culture, and the concomitant overvaluing of the intellect. Stone and Winkelman extended this idea and recognize disowned selves of all kinds.

The disowned self is an energy pattern that has been partially or totally excluded from one's life. It is an energy pattern that has been punished in the past every time it has emerged. These punishments may have been subtle or more powerful, like physical or psychological beating. In order for the subject to survive, the Primary Selves in collaboration with the Inner Critic had to exclude these energy patterns from the person's life. They were deemed totally unacceptable and were repressed, but not totally destroyed. These energy patterns remain alive in the unconscious.

From a Jungian perspective, the disowned selves comprise a part of our shadow. When we meet other people in our lives that carry these disowned energy patterns, our corresponding internal energies begin to vibrate; they cause a feeling of discomfort, for they are related to painful experiences that we had in the past. In such situations, the most common way to stop the vibrations of the disowned energy patterns is to judge the other person.

There is an important distinction between a disowned self and an undeveloped self. The generic term for a self that is not conscious is an unconscious self. Not all unconscious selves are necessarily disowned; some can be undeveloped.

For example, there is a part of us that has to do with being a parent. As long as we don't have children, this part is simply undeveloped. It is not disowned, for no energy is involved in holding it down. On the other hand, every disowned self has an opposite energy, with which the Ego and the Primary Selves are identified. This opposite energy, in conjunction with the Primary Selves, constantly holds the disowned self at bay.

A good way to find out about our disowned selves is to observe our reactions to and judgements about other people. If someone causes a strong reaction of repulsion and judgement in us, it is very likely that this person triggers one of our disowned selves. It is important to find out which particular characteristic evokes our reaction. What sort of energies are involved?

If, for example, someone has disowned his sexuality, goes to a party and enters a room where there is another person for whom the sexual energy is totally present, the disowned sexuality in the first person will begin to vibrate in sympathy, but at the same time the old pains will be felt again. The easiest way for this person to stop this annoying feeling is to judge the person for whom sexual energy is totally present. These phenomena can happen between two people without any evident action taking place. The energy bodies pick up the disowned frequencies quite accurately.

If people have done some Voice Dialogue transformational work and have developed an awareness level and a more Aware Ego, they can explore for themselves the energy pattern that is holding down the disowned self, and they may be able to let the disowned self be dialogued in a session. The session can both release the energy that was involved in holding it down and allow the energy of the formerly disowned self to be owned. In this way, the transformation of that disowned energy takes place.

III: Ego

At the level of the ego, transformation occurs when the ego disidentifies from whatever subpersonality dominates it, to an Aware Ego that has access to a far greater number of energy patterns. An ego that has such access is known as an empowered ego. That is, an empowered ego is an ego that has awareness of, and access to, both our powerful side and our vulnerable side and, therefore, is in a position to make *real* choices. In this way, we are not prisoners of the bonding patterns that happen between our energies and the energies of those around us. Although the bonding patterns happen, because the process is archetypal, we have the option of communicating from an Aware Ego level, thus stepping out of the bonding.

The consciousness model differs from other philosophical and religious traditions in that Awareness, Experience of Energy Patterns, and Ego are all represented, whereas, in eastern and western esoteric teachings, consciousness is usually defined as awareness. This traditional definition of consciousness as awareness causes a mind-body split.

The more traditional the religion, the more emphasis on the mind-body split. Stone and Winkelman observed that the same thing is happening in the New Age movement. Striving for more awareness can be used as an escape from experiencing such undesired energies as jealousy, pain, anger, so that these energies are made to go underground, into the unconscious. When the escape from undesired energies is legitimized by a philosophical tradition, awareness can be used as an alibi by the Inner Critic. Our Inner Critics love such ideas.

In Humanistic Psychology (i.e., in Gestalt, Bioenergetics and neo-Reichian work), it was important to integrate the emotions and the body.

In Transpersonal Psychology, on the other hand, the Awareness level is particularly emphasized; from this perspective people may easily confuse the state of Awareness with the experience of tranquility, harmony and peace.

In the consciousness model, peace and tranquility are viewed as energy patterns, along with other possible experiences. According to the Stone-Winkelman model, every experience can be accepted as long as the Awareness follows it, and we don't become overly identified with it.

The process of becoming aware and experiencing the energy patterns quite naturally diminishes the power of the so-called "Primary Selves," such as the Inner Critic, the Perfectionist, and nowadays the New Age "Spiritual Pusher."

VOICE DIALOGUE

DESCRIPTION OF METHOD AND GUIDELINES

In the Voice Dialogue method, Awareness, Experience of Energy Patterns, and Ego all have their own respective places.

Stone and Winkelman developed the Voice Dialogue method organically, in their own relationship, as a means to communicate with each other on different levels. As they describe it:

> *This method is called Voice Dialogue, which we developed as a means of working with one another psychologically when we first met in the early seventies. We felt that we needed some new tool to help us in our transformational processes, one that would help us to move beyond our own rational, intuitive, and psychologically sophisticated Primary Selves, and would encourage an ever widening expansion of consciousness. (Stone and Winkelman, 1985, p. 36)*

The method and the guidelines Stone and Winkelman give for the facilitator are as follows:

BASIC COMPONENTS

1) Exploration of Subpersonalities and Energy Systems

The facilitator engages in a dialogue with the different subpersonalities or archetypes. Each of them gets a separate physical space, e.g., chair, sofa, pillow, so that each can be objectified and separated out, without the interference of other subpersonalities or the Ego.

Each subpersonality is addressed directly, with full recognition of both its individual importance and its role as only a part of the total personality. Each subpersonality or archetype is a distinct energy pattern that animates the physical body with its own particular energies. The subject experiences this from the inside, whereas, the facilitator tunes in to the energies of the subject and observes changes that occur in order to help the subject move to a different place if another subpersonality takes over. The basic idea of the work is that of a joint exploration, not problem-solving or goal-seeking.

2) Clarification of Ego

Secondly, Voice Dialogue separates the Ego from the Primary Selves and the dominant subpersonalities that work alongside it. The Ego is given its own central physical space, and the subpersonalities play out their conflicts around it. When a subpersonality begins to take over the Ego, the alert Voice Dialogue facilitator will point out this takeover, will ask the subject to move to another space, and will then engage the new subpersonality directly. In this way, the Ego becomes more and more clearly differentiated; it becomes a more Aware Ego.

3) Enhancement of Awareness

Last of all, Voice Dialogue introduces Awareness into the system. There is a physical space for each subpersonality that does the experiencing, there is physical space for the Ego, who coordinates and executes, and there is physical space, separate from all the others, for Awareness. The space for Awareness is usually standing behind the Ego space. After having worked with different parts, the subject goes to this place and the facilitator reviews the session briefly and objectively. The subject remains silent and, from this still point, witnesses all that is going on, in a non-judgemental way, with no decisions to make.

GUIDELINES FOR THE FACILITATOR
(Stone and Winkelman, 1985, pp. 42-55)

1) Identification of Energy Patterns.
2) Physical separation of subpersonalities.
3) The facilitator takes the subpersonalities as real people. The attitude should be one of acceptance and empathy.
4) Separating the subpersonalities from the ego. This may require some intervention from the facilitator.
5) Remain non-judgemental and accepting.
6) Relax and take your time.
7) Observing changes in the Energy Patterns in order to move to different subpersonalities.
8) Voice Dialogue can induce altered states of consciousness. The facilitator should be aware of this possibility and protect the subject against any outside interventions.
9) Voice Dialogue is not to be used as a substitute for personal reactions. These reactions should be dealt with first, before starting a session; there should be no hidden agendas.

BUILT-IN PROTECTION

The built-in protection of the work is characterized by the fact that the Primary Selves are fully honored. No attempts are made to push people into new and different experiences, and no attempts are made to slip past the Primary Selves. The name Primary Selves already honors their protective function. This posture sounds a lot more positive than the usual "resistance."

It is this honoring of the Primary Selves that makes the work safe. Their function has been and still is the protection of our vulnerability. They make sure that we don't get into a new psychological arena too soon. When they give their permission to explore "new" energy patterns, the changes that occur in the subject's energy system are usually permanent and will not be followed by the reappearance of the angry Primary Selves that had been shoved underground.

This leads to a harmonious and balanced unfolding of our different parts or selves. Once the Primary Selves begin to trust the work and the transformational process, safe expeditions into new territory can begin. Although the developing Aware Ego has disidentified from the Primary Selves, it still values its protective function and considers its opinion in the choices that we make in our lives.

3

ENERGY

The fact that the concept of energy is used more and more in psychological work is due both to recent developments in modern physics, and to growing interest in "healing," eastern philosophy, and systems like Yoga and T'ai Chi Ch'uan. Modern physics has confirmed the ideas of the old Greek philosopher Heraclitus that everything is in a constant flow—panta rei. Solid matter does not exist, everything is built up of subatomic particles, and our environment is saturated with numerous kinds of radiation. In addition to ordinary visible light, there exist X-rays, gamma rays, infrared heat, ultra-violet light, radio waves, and cosmic rays. Lama Govinda, describing the Tibetan Buddhist view of consciousness as being composed of several shades, bands or levels, states that these levels "are not separate layers...but rather in the nature of mutually penetrating forms of energy, from the first all-radiating, all-pervading luminous consciousness down to the densest form of materialized consciousness, which appears before us as our visible, physical body." Kushi gives a clear explanation of eastern philosophy and eastern medicine, acupuncture, and macrobiotics.

Tao, the Chinese word denoting the order of the universe, creates the opposite forces Yin (negative) and Yang (positive), that in endless combinations and variations create energy and all visible and invisible phenomena. One of these energies is known as Ki, Chi, or Prana, the life force that penetrates our body like an electromagnetic field along the so-called meridians.

Western scientific research about Chinese acupuncture can be found in Krippner and Rubin.

In paraphysics, a science that studies the physics of paranormal processes, much research has been done on the electromagnetic fields of living organisms. Burr, who had already developed his theory in 1938, went on to develop, together with Ravitz and Northrop, instruments to measure electromagnetic fields that would confirm the theory. He concluded that these fields are everywhere and that they are prerequisite for, and determine the behavior of, matter.

In 1962, the Russian Vasiliev published his theory about the "mental fields" that play a role in telepathy. The Russian research also confirms the analogy between psychic energy, which the Russians call bioplasm, and electric energy. Kirlian became well known by photographing this energy, the so-called "aura photography." Western research on Kirlian photography is also considered in Krippner and Rubin.

All this recent research, Russian and otherwise, confirms the ideas of eastern and esoteric traditions about the nature of matter and consciousness and also confirms the perceptions of clairvoyants and mystics.

BODY ENERGY FIELDS OR AURA

The aura, also referred to as energy fields, was defined by the late W.E. Butler, a well-known English clairvoyant and the leader of a Western esoteric school, in the following way:

A subtle and invisible essence of fluid that emanates from human or animal bodies and even from things, a psychic electro-vital and electro-mental effluvium, partaking of both mind and body. (Butler, 1971, p. 7)

In clairvoyant vision, the aura is usually seen as a luminous atmosphere around all living things, including what used to be regarded as inanimate matter. Scientific research proves that, even in this so-called "dead" matter, living forces are at work. In this respect, Butler mentions that this research is "supporting the old Persian poet who wrote of life as 'sleeping in the mineral, dreaming in the plant, awakening in the animal and becoming conscious of itself in man'."

Occultists claim that the human aura consists of four different layers or energy "bodies"—the etheric, the emotional, the mental, and the spiritual body.

The etheric body is believed to control the metabolic processes of the physical body. The etheric body also draws vital energy (Prana, Ki, Chi) from the sun, and other forms of energy from the earth itself, for use in the living economy of the body cells. These energies circulate throughout the etheric body and its dense material counterpart, and, having supplied the needs of the organism, they are radiated out from the physical body in a peculiar haze which extends all around the body for some inches beyond its surface. This haze is known as the etheric aura. Since it is so closely connected with all the vital processes of the body, the appearance that the etheric aura presents to a clairvoyant healer is usually a good guide to the physical health of the person concerned. For this reason, diagnosis by the aura is a widespread practice in occult circles.

When we refer to the emotional, mental and spiritual bodies, the term "body" may be somewhat misleading. These finer bodies are best described as "vehicles" or "sheaths" (koshas).

Although most occult schools, in their practices, differentiate between the "emotional" and the "mental" bodies, these "bodies" are often intertwined, just as emotions and thought are closely linked together. The energies of the inner worlds of emotion and thought stream through these "bodies," which are our means of contact with those worlds. These energies also radiate out around the physical body, but over a far larger area than the vital energies of the etheric body. Whereas the extent of those vital radiations can usually be reckoned in inches, the combined emotional-mental radiation extends for several feet in the average person, and in more highly developed people it may extend even farther.

The spiritual aura, finally, is said to extend beyond the physical body, varying from a few feet, in the case of unevolved people, to yards or even miles, in the case of highly developed people. According to Butler, it is said in the East that the spiritual aura of the Buddha extended for two hundred miles and that the whole of this planet is held in the aura of a very great Being. The Christian teaching is similar, though it is usually restricted to the presence of the Deity. "In Him we live and move and have our being," as St. Paul says. It will be clear from this discussion that there is not one aura but several auras, each with its own peculiarities, working together as a composite atmosphere surrounding a person and serving as a part of the flow of inner energies through all parts of the being. These energy fields constantly reflect the general emotional and mental quality of our consciousness, and, due to the emotional and mental habits that we have developed, this general quality is relatively stable. The result is a certain general coloring for each person's aura, which furnishes a clairvoyant with a clear indication of the emotional, mental and spiritual character of the aura's owner.

THE CHAKRAS OR CENTERS

As already mentioned, the western esoteric tradition, of which W.E. Butler was part, teaches that the etheric body draws energy from the sun and from the earth as well.

There are certain points within the etheric body, all located along the spinal column, through which this dual stream of vitality is passed into the physical body. These distribution points are usually termed chakras (the Sanskrit term for wheels). To a clairvoyant, the chakras look like whirlpools or trumpet-shaped vortices of energy, and where the vortices touch the outer edge of the aura, they are covered by what looks like a fine and tenuous web of etheric substance. The vortices are constantly in a spinning motion, and, according to the direction of their spin, the energy appears to be drawn in or radiated out.

In addition to its function of distribution of vital energy from the etheric body into the physical body, each chakra is considered the center of a different psychophysical function.

The following overview of the chakras and their corresponding psychological functions is based on Brugh Joy's description:

1) The first chakra, the root center, an area one to three inches in diameter, is centered in the perineum, between the anus and the genitals. This center has to do with physicality and survival.

2) The second chakra, an area two to four inches in diameter, is centered in the lower abdomen above the pubic bone but below the navel. It is considered the sexual chakra.

3) The third chakra is located on the solar plexus, an area an inch and a half to four inches in diameter, centered in the pit of the stomach approximately two inches below where the ribs come together. This center is connected to power and emotions.

4) The fourth center is the heart chakra, an area an inch and a half to four inches in diameter, located above the place where the ribs come together on the lower front part of the chest. This center is related to unconditional love and love for mankind.

5) The fifth chakra is the throat chakra, an area an inch and a half to three inches in diameter, just above the junction of the collarbones. This center is considered the center of communication and creativity.

6) The sixth chakra is the brow or forehead center, an area an inch and a half to two inches in diameter, around the center of the forehead just above the level of the eyebrows. This center relates to our mental and psychic functioning.

7) The seventh chakra, or the crown center, is an area two to three inches in diameter around the center of the head. Here is our connection to the divine, feelings of total harmony are related to this center.

In addition to the seven major centers, there are centers located in the hands, elbows, shoulders, knees, feet, hips, upper chest and spleen. Besides these areas, where the energy fields are relatively strong, there are subtler areas of radiation all over the body.

ENERGY WORK

There have always been people who see auras and work with the body energy fields in order to heal or manipulate the energies of other people. In the last fifteen years, the interest in workshops like "aura healing" and "chakra balancing" has grown enormously in the West. The work of Brugh Joy and Carolyn Conger is well known in the New Age movement. They developed several techniques like scanning of body energy fields in order to diagnose which areas needed more attention. They also send healing energy through their hands to the afflicted areas. These techniques and others are described in Brugh Joy's book, *Joy's Way*. An important basis for the work is the fact that energy can be directed, expressed in the maxim that *energy follows thought*.

Most "healers" emphasize the fact that they are a "channel" for healing energies coming from God (or Source, as Carolyn Conger calls it). They open themselves to Source, and energy enters the body through the seventh chakra and flows through their hands to the afflicted areas of the person they are healing. Such channeling of energy can be done not only with individuals but also in group work

Another important axiom in the work is that energy is *inductive*. Many people experience this phenomenon in nature, feeling nurtured by a tree or by a rock. In this respect, Carolyn Conger, during a seminar in the Netherlands, told us about experiments that tested the effect of mud on hyperactive children and demonstrated that the slow vibratory pulsations of the mud had a soothing effect on the children. Healers and energy workers use this principle of induction, for example, by opening the heart chakra to radiate unconditional love. From this principle, it follows that it is important to be aware of our own energies as they influence other people.

The principle of induction is closely related to the principle of *resonance*. In the same way that a sound is reinforced and prolonged by the reflection of vibration of other bodies, our aura and chakras are affected by others. To state it in another way, the energy patterns of one person start to vibrate in sympathy with the same energy patterns of another person or object.

Another axiom is that *energy is neutral*. Whether we experience energy as good or bad has nothing to do with the energy and everything to do with ourselves and our perceptions.

An important technique worth mentioning in healing work is *shielding*, which is also utilized a great deal in native American traditions. By imagining a protective shield, brick wall or crystal bowl around oneself, one can protect oneself from unwanted surrounding energies. This exercise is based on the axiom that energy follows thought. In the same respect, one can consciously extend one's energy fields. Trained energy workers usually have a high level of awareness of the activities of their own energy fields, and in interactions with other people, they notice on which energy levels there is an exchange of energy and on which levels there is apparently no interaction.

For specific exercises and applications of working with body energy fields and the chakras that can be incorporated into Voice Dialogue training, see the Appendix.

T'AI CHI CH'UAN

My work with T'ai Chi Ch'uan over the last few years has encompassed working with several masters of the art, especially Dr. Kwee Swan Ho and Master Benjamin Lo. Master Benjamin Lo, originally from Taiwan, now has a school in San Francisco, and Dr. Ho carries on his work in Amsterdam. The T'ai Chi Ch'uan practice is based on basic principles that are not merely philosophical or theoretical but have been critically tested in combat over centuries. These principles will be seen to be valuable for psychological work and transformation of consciousness.

"T'ai Chi" is the popular abbreviation for T'ai Chi Ch'uan. The symbol of the eternal Tao is actually called T'ai Chi, meaning "the supreme ultimate" or "the grand terminus." The symbol is composed of a circle divided into two parts, called Yin and Yang, that are harmoniously interconnected. It signifies everything that is manifested in creation and the polarity that is contained in all. The word "Ch'uan" means fist or fighting system. This T'ai Chi Ch'uan can be defined as the supreme ultimate system of boxing or martial art.

Although the origins of Tai Chi Ch'uan are not clear, it is generally believed to have been developed by Taoist monks, who, in ancient China, had to defend themselves. Trying to translate their principles of philosophy and meditation into kinesthetic and energetic principles, they began experimenting and gradually evolved a highly sophisticated martial art that, more recently, has gained popularity in the West. The T'ai Chi form is a series of slow movements, done in a fluid, concentrated way, like a beautiful measured dance. The movements massage the internal organs and stimulate meridian lines and acupressure points, promoting health and well-being.

The T'ai Chi principles embody a deep mental and physical *relaxation* that is at the same time alert and anticipatory.

The body relearns to connect to earth energies and to the higher energies; this connection is known as *alignment.* Movement is always made from an inseparable mental and physical *center,* and the practitioner learns to work with the *Yin-Yang Principle* by becoming aware of the opposing forces in the body and balancing them. By practicing the form in his way, remarkable changes occur in the body and the energy flow. In China, T'ai Chi is used as a preventive and curative system of medicine.

Indeed, the first result for the practitioner is an increased health and sense of well-being and a greater awareness of one's own energy system. After mastering the form, the next step is the so-called "push hands" practice, where two people practise together. In this practice, one also learns to become sensitive to other people's energies, to *yield* to these energies without losing one's center, and to direct one's energy. In the push-hands practice, participants test each other's skills, and thus help each other to become aware of areas of their practice that needs more attention.

Eventually, after many years, people can develop remarkable skills. In China, there are numerous stories of old men easily and successfully fighting many young men. Some T'ai Chi masters are also renowned healers, a few of whom are said to heal broken bones instantly.

What all T'ai Chi masters stress is that it is of no use to practice T'ai Chi, even for many years, without following its principles. These principles are described in "The T'ai Chi Classics." A proper understanding of the T'ai Chi principles, however, cannot be obtained from reading but only by prolonged practice under the guidance of a master of the tradition who embodies the teachings of the T'ai Chi Classics.

MAJOR PRINCIPLES OF T'AI CHI CH'UAN

1. Mind directs the Chi

Awareness can be focused on various parts of the body and its movements, causing a change in energy experience and a change in the quality of the energy.

The mind mobilizes the Chi. Make the Chi sink calmly, then it gathers and permeates the bones. The chi mobilizes the body. Make it move smoothly, then it easily follows (the direction of) the mind. (Master Wu Yu-hsiang, in Lo, et al.)

It is interesting to note how closely this principle of T'ai Chi relates to the first axiom of the aforementioned healing tradition: *energy follows thought*.

2. Relaxation

The body and mind need to be relaxed in order for the Chi to circulate freely.

In practising T'ai Chi Ch'uan the whole body relaxes. Don't let one ounce of force remain in the blood vessels, bones and ligaments to tie yourself up. Then you can be agile and able to change. You will be able to turn freely and easily. Doubting this, how can you increase your power? The body has meridians like the ground has ditches and trenches. If not obstructed, the water can flow. If the meridian is not closed, the Chi goes through. If the whole body has hard force and it fills up the meridians, the Chi and the blood stop and the turning is not smooth and agile. (Chen Wei-ming, Commentary on Yang Cheng-fu's Ten Important Points, in Lo, et al., 1979, p. 87)

3. Alignment

The third principle, alignment, comes from the Taoist idea of Man between Heaven and Earth. In the body, alignment is expressed by straightening the spine, dropping the shoulders and chest and relaxing the abdomen in order to let the Chi sink downward to the soles of the feet, while at the same time, the top of the head should be suspended. One should imagine a line through the body connecting earth and heaven. By letting the weight drop completely, giving it to the earth, energy will come back from the earth into the body. Through the top of the head energy can come in as well.

Completely relax the abdomen and the Chi rises up. When the coccyx is straight, the (shen) spirit goes through to the headtop. To make the whole body light and agile suspend the headtop. (Unknown author, in Lo, et al.)

4. Move from Center

The fourth principle is to move from center. The Chi is stored in the *tantien* an area two inches below the navel. From there, the Chi is distributed throughout the body and can be directed to the hands and legs. Every movement starts from the waist; the hands and legs follow.

The waist is the commander of the whole body. If you can relax the waist, then the two legs will have power and the lower part will be firm and stable. Substantial and insubstantial change, and this is based on the turning of the waist. (Chen Wei-ming, in Lo, et al)

5. The Yin-Yang principle

In the T'ai Chi tradition, man is a dynamic energy system made up of the opposite forces of Yin and Yang. T'ai Chi consciously accentuates this polarity in order to increase the energy flow between Yin and Yang, which results in a better health and more internal force.

The main way to "stretch" the Yin and Yang polarity in T'ai Chi is to focus on the division of the weight in the legs while making the movements. At any moment, the leg that carries the body's weight is called the Yang, or full, and the leg that has no weight on it is called Yin, or empty. When we walk normally, the shifting of the weight goes quite quickly, so that the fluctuation of Yin and Yang, with regular intervals, may hardly be noticed. In T'ai Chi practice, however, the movements are made very slowly, with slightly bent legs, while the upper body is relaxed. By moving in this way, more weight can sink into each leg. The time spent on each pole is now longer and the intensity greater than when we walk normally. This "stretching" of the Yin and Yang poles produces an increase of the energy flow between the two polarities. Because many meridians end in the soles of our feet, our whole energy system is affected.

This principle of stretching the Yin and Yang is of vital importance in T'ai Chi and is maintained throughout all the movements. It not only differentiates between full and empty legs, but also between the upper and lower parts of the body and between areas to which more or less Chi is directed. During the movements, there is a constant stretching and fluctuating of the Yin and Yang. This principle is the motor of the Chi flow and is described in many tests, as for example:

Stand like a balance and
Rotate actively like a wheel.
Sinking to one side is sluggish
Being double-weighted is sluggish.

Anyone who spent years of practice
and still cannot neutralize,
and is always controlled by his opponent,
has not apprehended
the fault of double-weightedness.

To avoid this fault
one must know Yin and Yang

Yin and Yang
mutually aid and change each other.
(Wang Tsung-yueh, in Lo et al.)

The five principles described are closely interrelated and therefore should be interpreted in relation to each other. The more one can concentrate, relax, be aligned and move from the waist, the more the Yin and Yang will be differentiated, resulting in a stronger and more vital energy flow.

For specific exercises that demonstrate the T'ai Chi Ch'uan principles and can be incorporated into the Voice Dialogue training, see the Appendix.

4

THE ENERGETICS OF
VOICE DIALOGUE

As has been stated, the tradition of Voice Dialogue is fundamentally based on the knowledge that we are made up of different parts or energy patterns.

These parts are recognized, real, and unique in themselves. They can think, express themselves, have their own feelings, and they can feel good or angry towards the ego, depending on how the ego treats them. In this study, the most important emphasis is on their relationships to the physical body and its energy fields.

For example, a subpersonality like the Rational Controller will very likely be related to the head area but may also have a particular connection to the chest and breathing function. It will also relate to particular areas of the aura and the chakra system.

Compared to the Rational Controller, a Vulnerable Child subpersonality will have a very different physical presence, which will be expressed, not just in the facial area, but in the whole body. In addition, the chakras can be observed to begin to vibrate differently when a person moves into the Vulnerable Child energy pattern.

Although the Awareness level simply witnesses and is not part of the energy patterns, it does have an impact on the experience of energy patterns.

In Voice Dialogue, we don't work directly with the physical body and the energy fields as in the esoteric healing traditions and T'ai Chi Ch'uan, but here, the axiom that *energy follows thought,* results in a deeper experience of the subpersonalities or energy patterns. When the awareness is brought to certain parts of ourselves as the parts are objectified in a Voice Dialogue session, the experience of their energy will change and become more intense. The flow of psychic energy will go to the part on which the awareness focuses.

As pointed out earlier, the facilitator's job is to help the subject separate the different subpersonalities or energy patterns, help him clarify the ego, and facilitate the Awareness level.

Because the parts have an energetic quality with a way of expressing themselves, the facilitation is an interplay of verbal and energetic communication.

It is important to note that the transformational quality of the work is not due to analysis and rational understanding. Therefore, it is paramount that the facilitator not be identified with his rational mind. Although the rational mind can be very useful in the work, and the facilitator and subject can benefit from its ideas, it is just one among many energy patterns, and the facilitator should be able to switch it on and off at will; otherwise, it may arrest the dialogue process by keeping it on a strictly mental level. In some cases, it may even interfere with the dialogue process, e.g., when the facilitator is talking to a non-rational part of the subject, like the Freedom voice or the Sensual part. These voices will most likely be disturbed by rational questions that don't match the energy.

Obviously, for the facilitator, Voice Dialogue is quite a sophisticated training on various levels. He is trained to maintain an awareness of both the subject's energies and the changes and fluctuations in his own energy patterns as a result of the work. As he experiences more energy patterns in the course of his work, he becomes more capable of *resonating* with and *inducting* a wider variety of energy patterns so that he can facilitate ever more subtle levels of consciousness.

The facilitator has to maintain a balance between going along with the energies and keeping his Awareness present. From the Aware Ego vantage point, the experienced facilitator is in a position to make the appropriate choices in the work to facilitate the subject's transformational process.

The Voice Dialogue axiom, "Consciousness is the awareness and experience of energy patterns," can best be clarified by actually moving through the consecutive phases in an average Voice Dialogue session.

PHASE ONE: THE EGO SPACE

The facilitator and the subject sit facing each other. The subject's place is called the Ego Space. The exact place to sit should be chosen with awareness. Before actually beginning the session, the facilitator senses whether he and the subject are sitting in the right spot, whether the distance between him and the subject feels right or they should move closer or farther apart. The energetically aware facilitator will be able to find his "power spot," the working place that is in harmony with all the surrounding energies. Since others' energy fields can affect the session, it is important, if there are observers, to sense whether they are sitting at the right place and distance. This preparation is very important.

The facilitator now takes a moment to *center*: he *relaxes*, lets go of mental activity, brings his attention to his body, and lets go of tensions. He consciously connects with the earth and *aligns* himself to heaven, or higher energies, so that he can become a *channel* for healing energies.

Once the facilitator begins the session, he is both energeticaly aware of what is going on, and communicating verbally. He may ask whether there is an area that the subject wants to explore in the session, and they may spend a period of time in the Ego Space discussing the issue to be addressed before they begin the work of separating out subpersonalities from the Ego.

On an energetic level, the energy fields of subject and facilitator are already merging, in the sense that even before a word is said, the various layers of the aura and the chakras of subject and facilitator will begin to vibrate together.

In this way, the energetically aware facilitator gets information about the subject. To enhance this process, he consciously *opens himself energetically* and makes himself receptive. He listens with an inner ear to what goes on with the energies. The principle involved here is that of *resonance*: the energy patterns of the facilitator start to resonate with those of the subject. Consequently, the facilitator can *scan* the energies of the subject.

The Voice Dialogue facilitator uses two basic ways of scanning. With the first, he starts by sensing what is happening in his own body and energy fields as a result of resonating with the subject. He may notice that a particular area of his body is starting to feel tense and contracted. If he has done sufficient transformational work himself and the tension is not caused by a disowned self of his own, the reaction provides valuable information about the subject. If he tunes in to the tense area, he may get in touch with certain feelings or emotions, like sadness or anger, and so, he may get an idea of the subpersonalities of the subject that can be worked with. The facilitator may also notice areas of the body or certain chakras that are particularly vibrant and alive, reflecting other subpersonalities of the subject that can be engaged in a dialogue.

In the second way of scanning, the facilitator consciously checks in on his own subpersonalities and brings them forward energetically to feel how they react to the subject's energy patterns. This internal operation happens in quite a subtle way and may be hardly noticed by the subject.

By checking in with his own vulnerability aspect or inner Child, the facilitator can get information on the state of the subject's inner Child. As he focuses on his own inner Child and allows it to come forward, its energy will manifest in his body and energy fields: *energy follows thought.* The facilitator's inner Child will know whether the subject's inner Child is available and how it feels emotionally, e.g., sad, happy, hurt, playful.

Since the energetic vibration of the inner Child is probably the finest and most sensitive of all our energy patterns, it is important for the Voice Dialogue facilitator's inner Child to be available. It connects us not, only to nature in its widest sense, but also to our own essence, and it is, therefore, the window to our soul. It is the aspect that makes real contact with another person possible.

In the same way that the facilitator can consciously connect with his inner Child, he can check in with his inner Warrior, or some other subpersonality that carries his particular instinctual energies, such as an animal form like a tiger, snake, or dragon. Such an energy pattern will sense if the subject's instinctual energies are available or if they have been disowned. Having these instinctual energies at his disposal will help the facilitator avoid getting locked into a form and enable him to move with what is present in the moment.

As the facilitator engages with the subject, his own energy patterns, such as the Child and the Warrior, should be available without dominating the session. They are like actual energy bodies surrounding us that can be invited in or asked to withdraw.

The fact that the energy patterns are really energy bodies with a particular relation to the Ego Space is fascinating. The experienced energetic facilitator can sometimes detect the energy bodies of the subject even before a session has started. He may sense an area in the room a few feet from the subject that seems to pull in the subject's energies.

Needless to say, in order to work in this energetic way, the facilitator must have a well-developed Aware Ego. That is, he needs an overall awareness of energy patterns, both inside himself and around himself, and, in this connection, he needs to be aware of the axiom that *energy follows thought* and to embody the T'ai Chi principles of *alert relaxation, alignment,* and being *centered.*

In this first phase, engaging with the subject in the Ego Space, it is also important for the facilitator to recognize the prevailing energy, the energy pattern or patterns with which the subject is identified. When moving toward Phase Two, in which a part is separated from the Ego, the facilitator is advised not to go against the prevailing energy but rather to go with it by talking to that part first. This choice may differ from the subject's perception of what should be done. It is important for the facilitator not to get hooked into what the subject says, and so lose a clear perspective on the state of the energy patterns.

In Voice Dialogue sessions, there is often a subpersonality of the subject that likes to make agendas. This subpersonality is usually a "cluster" of Controller, Pusher and Inner Critic operating as a unit at the beginning of the work. This cluster subpersonality often works in all aspects of the subject's life, so that making an agenda for the Voice Dialogue session is simply a natural procedure for it. It may want the subject to work with anger and aggression and to re-experience this or that trauma, all in one session. If the subject is overly identified with this voice, he will ask the facilitator to work on the anger, the aggression, and the trauma.

If the facilitator operates from a predominantly mental perspective, he will be unable to identify this cluster energy pattern in the subject and will get hooked by what the subject says. Thus, he will *lose his center* and a clear perspective on the state of the energy patterns. From a clear perspective, words and ideas are just energy patterns. If, in this example, the facilitator loses his center, the subject's cluster will run the session, and it is unlikely that any real transformational work will be accomplished.

In such a situation, one way to work without losing one's center, and without offending the subject, is to suggest talking to the voice that made the agenda for the session. In this way, the cluster's prevailing energy will be separated out from the Ego and engaged directly in the second phase. This approach is related to the T'ai Chi principle of *yielding*, in which the facilitator yields to the prevailing energy so that it is honored and may be explored.

PHASE TWO: SEPARATING OUT AN ENERGY PATTERN

The energetically aware facilitator will now be in a position to make a conscious choice about the first energy pattern to be objectified in the session, based on the data he has gathered in Phase One.

The facilitator now asks the subject to move to a different physical space to allow the part or subpersonality to separate itself. On a verbal level, the facilitator makes his acquaintance with the part as if it were a new person he has just met and invites it to communicate. By asking what the part thinks, feels, or likes to do, he will elicit valuable information for the Awareness level and the Ego level of the subject.

Energetically, several things happen. When the subject has moved from the Ego Space to the space of the subpersonality, the facilitator first *opens himself energetically*, takes a moment to feel the particular energy of the part, to feel which areas of his energy body *resonate* with it. After letting the energy in, the facilitator allows the corresponding part of himself to come forward and *drops into* it, so that that energy is really available for the facilitator in communicating with the subject's subpersonality. This will *induct* the subject more deeply into the experience of the particular energy pattern. While communicating energetically, the facilitator keeps his Awareness level operating so that he can detect energetic shifts and other parts or energies that may come in.

As the facilitator and the subject enjoy the same frequency, they both explore the energy for a while, going deeper and deeper into it. That is to say, the facilitator will have available in the communication an energy that is of the same nature, character, and strength, so that it induces the subject more deeply into the experience of the pattern. In relation to the pattern, however, the facilitator need not have the same subjective emotional experiences as the subject. For example, when the vulnerable Child of the subject experiences fear or anguish because it has been disowned for a long time, the facilitator's inner Child need not feel the same fear and anguish; rather, it can simply be present as a soft and vulnerable vibration that feels contact and connects with the subject's hurt Child.

When the facilitator has tuned in properly to the subpersonality and has *dropped into* the corresponding energy in himself, his voice and words will be fitting, so that the verbal aspect of the communication will also be based on the energetics. For example, in dialoguing with the Primary Selves, the facilitator will tune in to his own Primary Selves' energy and will be able to speak from there and use language and ask questions that will make sense to the subject's Protector-Controller.

The next thing to be aware of in the interaction, is that the energy will eventually begin to *diminish*. This will happen quite naturally, as every energy state has its limits and has an opposite energy that will be tending to pull from the other side of the polarity. I relate this to the *Yin-Yang principle* of T'ai Chi. When we have engaged the subpersonality in this energetic way and have gone fully, 100% into the experience of its energy, there will come a point where there will be a natural energy shift.

On a verbal level this shift may show by the subpersonality's having nothing more to say or repeating itself. On an energetic level, the facilitator will notice a decrease of the energy vibrations that are expressed in the voice, posture and energy body of the subject. The facilitator, of course, is aware of this change and is ready to follow the shift to another part.

PHASE THREE: MOVING TO THE NEXT PART

On the verbal level, the facilitator may suggest going to another part, or, if a new part is already manifesting, the facilitator may say something to the subject like: "Well, it seems that someone else is coming in. Perhaps we'd better talk to that part directly." The subject then moves to a different physical space in order to let the new part manifest fully.

The facilitator now lets go of the energy pattern in himself that was engaged in dialogue with the former part of the subject. That is, he lets go not only of the concepts, language structure, and perspective on life that it had, but also of its inherent physical posture and energetic vibration.

The facilitator consciously empties himself of all these contents by feeling his *center*, *relaxing* a moment, and *aligning* energetically with heaven and earth. This has a cleansing effect on his system and enables him to be refreshed to meet the new energy pattern.

He then goes again through the "movements" of *opening* to the new energy pattern, *resonating* with it, and then *dropping* into the corresponding energy in himself. If, for example, the new energy pattern is a Warrior, the facilitator lets his own Warrior come forward.

This process requires some skill. The facilitator's "Warrior energy" should manifest strong enough to induct and "hold" the subject's Warrior. It should not, however, manifest much stronger than the subject's energy pattern, because, if the subject is not yet familiar with the Warrior energy, the facilitator's too-strong Warrior may call forth the subject's Primary Selves. If, on the other hand, the facilitator correctly carries out the induction and "holding," the subject's Warrior will feel recognized and appreciated and will manifest more fully.

The induction of the Warrior energy pattern by the facilitator encompasses the holding of a stern physical posture and strong activity of his lower chakras, so that the instinctual energies can circulate freely and radiate outward from the facilitator's center. In this way, he will create and regulate a strong instinctual energy field around both himself and the subject. This energy field will induct the subject deeply into the experience of his own Warrior energy and make an in-depth exploration possible.

After exploring this energy state together for a while, there will come a moment when the energy shifts again. This shift is definitely an energetic experience. The facilitator may then suggest that the subject go back to the Ego Space. Or, if another part seems to present itself, he may suggest that the subject go to that new part, in which case the same procedures follow.

The number of energy patterns that are objectified in a session can vary—sometimes just one, usually two to four, sometimes four to eight.

PHASE FOUR: BACK TO THE EGO SPACE

The subject now moves back to the Ego Space in order to decide, together with the facilitator, whether or not to move on to the phase of Awareness, or whether to engage another energy pattern in dialogue to balance out the session.

In this phase, the subject usually has a pretty good sense of what needs to be done. The subject will have more awareness of the energy patterns that have manifested and will experience them more strongly in his body.

The facilitator will *scan* the subject's body and energy fields again, in the way that was described for Phase One. He can encourage the subject to bring his attention to certain areas of the body to check if they need more attention. The facilitator may scan in particular the areas that felt tense or contracted before the session began. Usually the body and energy field of the subject will feel quite differently from the way they felt in Phase One. When Voice Dialogue work is done from an energetic perspective, it tends to balance and harmonize the subject's energies.

Although there may always remain areas or energy patterns that need more work, the facilitator and subject will sense and "know" in this phase when they have reached the limit of what can be done in the session. The energy body of the subject will feel that this cycle of exploration has been accomplished.

PHASE FIVE: AWARENESS

The subject is now asked to go to the place of Awareness, which is usually designated as standing just behind the Ego Space, so that the full range of energy patterns that were explored in the session can now be witnessed.

The idea of standing in the place of Awareness is to invite the Awareness level to witness everything, from a detached and non-judgemental mode and without any effort to make an analysis of the session. The facilitator will then review the session objectively. He will point out the different energy patterns that manifested in the session and summarize what they said.

The full presence of the facilitator's Awareness will induct the Awareness level of the subject. In order to really invite the Awareness of the subject to be present, the facilitator will allow moments of silence between pointing out the various energy patterns.

In his review, the facilitator will pay special attention to the subject's physical and energetic experiences in the session. After describing a particular energy pattern and what it said, the facilitator can ask the subject to let that energy pattern be physically present in the place of Awareness.

As mentioned earlier, the different subpersonalities are really energy bodies that can be invited in or, likewise, asked to withdraw. Each energy body has its own physical place in relation to the subject. The facilitator can suggest that the subject invite an energy body in, experience its energetics, and then to let it go. Furthermore, he can suggest that the subject briefly re-experience as many energy bodies as have come out in a given session.

The review will allow the Awareness to fully *sink into* the various energy patterns, and be aware, not only of their mental contents, but also of their energetics and of the way they tend to pull on the ego from their respective places.

Usually, in the place of Awareness, the subject will experience some integration of the dynamic energies that have been explored. Also, certain insights relating to problem areas may be experienced at this time as the subject suddenly "sees" how things fall into place.

FINAL PHASE: GROUNDING THE EXPERIENCE

After being in the space of Awareness, the subject is asked to return to the Ego Space. In this Final Phase, the facilitator and subject can talk about the elements of the session. The subject may reflect on what has happened and discuss any thoughts that come up in relation to the session. The facilitator will ask whether the subject feels balanced and will again check this energetically through the techniques of *scanning* and *resonance*. Sometimes, in this Final Phase, little needs to be said. The time spent here is to ground the experience. The energetics of Voice Dialogue often *induct* people into altered states of consciousness, and it is important to allow time after a session so that the experiences can be integrated by the Ego. This integration can happen by talking with the facilitator or by just being quiet for a while.

It is also important that the facilitator prepare the subject to let go of the energetic connection that has developed between him and the subject. This connection is quite strong due to the energetic nature of the work. The energy fields of subject and facilitator have merged and their vital energies have circulated in harmony throughout the session. It is important for the facilitator not to break the connection abruptly but to prepare the subject verbally and then gently withdraw his energies. In this regard, he may suggest that the subject do a grounding exercise, in which the subject focuses on his own center, connects visually with the center of the earth, and invites higher energies to come in.

The facilitator is well advised to do the same thing himself, to let go of any energies that do not belong to him so that they won't stay in his aura. This is an important technique that is also used in the esoteric healing tradition. Once the subject feels grounded and balanced, the session can end.

SUMMARY OF ENERGETIC PRINCIPLES

As we have seen, the facilitator works on the three levels of the consciousness process—Awareness, Experience of Energy Patterns, and Ego. In order to perform at his optimum, he should not only follow the guidelines that were given at the end of Chapter 2, including such criteria as acceptance and a non-judgemental attitude, but also, in order to have an increased energetic proficiency, be prepared to practise the energetics principles that have been presented in this chapter.

Specific energetics principles for the facilitator that will enhance the facilitation are summarized below.

1)   An awareness of body and energy fields

This is necessary in order to tune in to the energies of the subject, notice energy shifts, and maintain the facilitator's awareness while he drops into a specific energy pattern in order to begin the dialogue process.

2)   Energy follows thought (Mind directs the Chi)

Through this principle, the facilitator can direct the flow of psychic energy to different parts of himself in order to induct the subject into different energy patterns.

3)   Resonance

By being aware of the energy patterns that start to resonate with those of the subject, the facilitator can scan the subject's energy patterns.

4)   Induction

By dropping into an energy pattern, the facilitator can induct the subject into experiencing this same energy pattern.

5)   Alert relaxation

An alert and anticipatory relaxation is a prerequisite to accomplish any of the above and to drop easily into energy patterns.

6)   Centeredness, physically and mentally
From a centered position, the facilitator can move with the energies of the subject without losing his psychological balance.

7)   Alignment with heaven and earth
By consciously aligning with the spaces of heaven and earth, the facilitator can be a channel for healing energy. He will be in a position to scan the subject's energy patterns that are related to the chakras.

8)   Awareness of the Yin-Yang Principle
While facilitating a subpersonality of the subject, the facilitator should also be aware of, and take into consideration, what might be going on at the other side of the energy spectrum. For example, if he is facilitating a power voice, he should be aware of his subject's vulnerability. The facilitator should be aware that when the energy has fully flown to one side of a polarity it will naturally shift to the other side of the polarity.

TWO EXAMPLES OF STRONG ENERGETICALLY BASED VOICE DIALOGUE SESSIONS

ALEX

The following case illustrates, step by step, the subtle movements in the energetics of the facilitation process. The case exemplifies an average Voice Dialogue session and will be described in detail to demonstrate the energetic principles in process.

On March 12, 1987, in one of my ongoing training groups, I had the following session with Alex, 45, the coordinator of a residential treatment center for adolescents. His work included the coordination of the treatment program and the financial organization of the center.

After experiencing a loss of energy in his work and private life, he had joined my group because he felt a need to do some personal transformational work. Before this session, one of my assistants had introduced him to the work and familiarized him with its concepts.

In the session, I first spent some time finding the right working place, and we then sat facing each other. Since Alex had a relatively strong energy field, I asked some of the observers to move back a little to allow enough working space.

After I sensed that we were sitting at the right place and at the right distance, I asked Alex to take a moment to bring his attention inward to focus on the issue he wanted to work with. While he did so, I took the time to center and empty myself of thoughts. From this centered position, I opened myself energetically for higher energies and visually connected with the center of the earth. With my position centered and aligned, I was aware of my own energy fields and chakras and felt them begin to resonate with those of Alex.

Since the circulation of vital energy through the energy fields and physical body is strongly connected to the breathing function, our breathing patterns were also aligned when our energy fields resonated in unison. With this alignment, I perceived that we were part of a larger energy field that resonated in unison. As a facilitator, I was receptive and followed the movements in his energy system in order to *scan* the state of his energies. What was evident to me in this phase, was the strong activity in Alex's head area and sixth chakra. I also noticed that his lower chakras were relatively closed in comparison to the higher ones.

When we started talking, I asked Alex whether there was an area in his life that he wanted to explore. He talked about his work and said that he often felt tired and drained. After we discussed his work situation briefly, it seemed evident to me that the prevailing energy in Alex, the energy that he was most identified with, was a very Rational Controller. I therefore suggested that he separate this energy pattern out in order to dialogue it.

Agreeing to my suggestions, Alex moved his chair a few feet to his right side and found a place that seemed to fit the energy pattern. I now opened myself energetically to the energy of his Rational Controller. Its main center was indeed the head and sixth chakra. As I tuned more into it, I allowed the corresponding part of myself to come forward, and I dropped into it. I let the rest of my energy patterns fade to the background, but I did not lose my awareness of them, for I knew they might give me information about possible energy shifts. The process of bringing my corresponding energy pattern forward encompassed a slight shift in my posture, so that I sat more straight and with increased tension in my upper body, especially the upper chest, neck, and shoulders. I also experienced a concentration of energy in my forehead and noticed increased activity in my sixth chakra. I felt that my corresponding energy pattern had to do with structure and keeping an overview of my activities. This entire maneuver, tuning in and dropping, took no more than one second.

As I now talked with Alex's Rational Controller, I let my correspond-ing energy pattern be present in the conversation. I asked the Rational

Controller what it did in Alex's life. Since the energy pattern felt invited by my induction, it manifested easily. It described itself as a controller. Its job was to take care of Alex's business and to provide structure in his life. It said that it was present most of the time. It had a crisp and clear energetic quality and seemed to do a lot of work for Alex. By asking many specific questions about its modus operandi, I elicited valuable information for the Awareness level that could later be processed by the Aware Ego, and I also went on to explore and "stretch" the energy pattern.

First, I explored how the Rational Controller operated for Alex in his personal life. It apparently made daily schedules for Alex, ranging from the letters it wanted him to write to making shopping lists. It also did long-term planning for Alex's career and development.

When I went on to explore how it was present in Alex's working situation, we reached a deeper level of the energy pattern. Through the principle of resonance, I experienced that his sixth chakra was now radiating more strongly and that his energy fields had expanded. The Rational Controller said that it was present in Alex's working situation in order to take care of the overall structure of the organization. As it went on to describe its activities in doing so, it seemed to take on a large archetypal energy. It stated that it kept track of organizational developments as well as the functioning of many staff members—all the various elements and structures that it had to handle and orchestrate. At this point in the conversation, it also said that it had an intuitive or psychic ability to detect any problems in the various levels of the organization.

By now, the energy had shifted slightly, but it was still the same energy pattern. It had been *stretched*, and I had gotten in touch with its "core," which I recognized as a truly Apollonian archetype. After a few minutes of rather abstract conversation about the nature of reality, the energy began to shift more noticeably.

Through the principle of resonance, I experienced a decrease of the energy, and I was also aware of a spot on the other side of Alex that seemed to pull on his energies. I then checked to see whether the Rational-Apollonian energy pattern had any more to say, and I then suggested Alex move to the other side to see who was there.

Alex then moved to a place at the left side of the Ego Space. As soon as he did so, his energies shifted totally. It was as if his weight had dropped and he experienced gravity for the first time. His head, neck and shoulders relaxed, and he started to breath deeply and slowly.

Letting go of the first energy pattern in myself, I made myself empty and receptive and, opening to the new part that manifested, I experienced a complete shift of energy. The physical center of the new part I perceived as being in the abdomen, and the lower chakras began to open. I allowed myself to sink into my own corresponding pattern in order to induce Alex further into it.

For a while, we said nothing. The energy pattern seemed very tired and needed time to relax. It was completely opposite from the previous part. When I allowed the corresponding part of myself to come forward, it was totally non-rational and couldn't care less about structure. From this inner space, I greeted the new part and just said, "Hi!" It raised its left hand and responded to my greeting with a low grunt. It seemed very weary. Gradually, by just being there and sinking into this space energetically, it started to talk. Its voice was about an octave lower, and the words came out slowly, right from the belly. Although the part was tired, I felt that it was quite powerful. It said something like: "Jesus Christ, this guy is nuts. Gimme a break... I'm fed up, really fed up, with this."

As I really took my time to just *be* with this part and allow it to feel its own energy, it somehow started to gain energy and speak more. It said that it really hated structures and couldn't care less about what happened in Alex's work. It just wanted to be there and "hang out." As I went on to explore it, it told me that it liked being with "the guys" and having a good time. At some point I experienced more sexual energy coming in, through a stronger vibration of the second chakra, and asked how it felt about women. Its grin became a devilish, Jack Nicholson smile, and it now became quite alive. It told me more about what it liked to do, given the chance.

Engaging this part released more and more energy and created a strong instinctual energy field in the room. We spent some time just being with this energy. The essence of the part, expressed in its own way, was a primordial energetic vibration that refused to be structured in any way. When the energy had manifested fully in Alex's body and energy fields, I again detected a shift.

The first thing I noticed was a different vibration in my heart chakra. As I tuned into Alex's heart chakra, I sensed that it had opened more. The instinctual energy now seemed to fade a bit, and I asked Alex to move a bit to his left, where I sensed that the new pattern was. The energy that now began to manifest had a very strong heart quality. When I resonated with it, I experienced a warm and "deep" feeling in my heart area. The energy with which I resonated had a wise feminine quality. I let my own corresponding energy come forward to induce the part of Alex that now manifested.

Alex's posture had changed; he sat in a relaxed manner, one leg over the other, and looked at me. When we spoke, the part described itself as an elegant woman. It said that it liked to sit on a terrace drinking a glass of wine and just watching people. It carried the feeling side of Alex and was very refined. The voice was soft and deep. It said that it could really connect with people's essence. It didn't have high ambitions in terms of achieving things in life. It enjoyed being there and would like to be there more. It also had some advice for Alex about his work and said that it could help him if he would allow space for it.

This part had a very soothing and healing energy, and the pattern itself felt very integrated and harmonious, qualities I experienced, not only in my heart chakra, but also in my whole energy field and body. After talking with it about its areas of interest, I suggested going back to the Ego Space, and it agreed. We had worked for about an hour. Back in the Ego Space, Alex and I both sensed energetically that it was time to end the session. When he moved to the place of Awareness, I reviewed the session, paying special attention to the energetic shifts that had taken place, so that he could witness and re-experience the energy patterns from this vantage point. In the Ego Space again, we discussed the session, and, after I had made sure that he felt balanced, we ended the session.

In summary, the session clearly demonstrated the natural process that takes place as a result of fully exploring the energy patterns. When one pattern has been fully "stretched" with the help of an energetically attuned facilitator, the energy will shift to the other side of the polarity. After Alex's Rational Controller was stretched, the instinctual energies manifested. After them, came yet another opposite polarity, of a nature different from the first one. By following and stimulating this natural flow through the energetics of the work, Alex restored his balance and gained vitality. The session proved to be an important breakthrough for Alex and helped him to find a new balance in his life. He began to disidentify from the Rational Controller and to embrace the instinctual, devilish side as well as the wise, feminine side.

CLAIRE

In the following case, the session began with a specific energetic focus in the sense that the client had a physiological complaint. By tuning in energetically to the problem area, the session proceeded through to a very dramatic conclusion.

On April 9, 1986, a young woman named Claire, a professional dancer, came to see me. For some time she had been experiencing a pressure in her chest that hindered her in performing, and she wanted me to do some energy work with her.

We sat facing each other and I asked her to bring her attention to her chest and breathe slowly. As I opened myself energetically to Claire and tuned in to the chest area, I felt my energies resonate with hers. Scanning in this way, I noticed a lot of tension in the chest area. For a while, she breathed slowly into the tense area and I resonated with her energetically, working from the heart chakra. The intensity of her energetic experience grew stronger until she suddenly experienced what appeared to be a jolt of energy, which shook her whole body so that she became very emotional and started to cry. I asked what had happened. Looking very shocked, she said that she had seen a very ugly, contorted, green face that had been haunting her in recurring nightmares for the last two years. I asked her whether she could keep her attention on the chest area and still allow that monstrous green face to stay present. Then, moving into a Voice Dialogue format, I asked whether I could speak to the green face. Claire said she would try. I asked her to move her chair a little bit.

When she had moved, I opened myself energetically to tune in to this particular energy vibration. It felt to me like a mixture of anger and agony, and I experienced a strong pressure in the chest area. Once I was aligned with the energy, resonating with the green monster, I "held" the energy in order to induce her deeper into the experience.

The green face seemed to be willing to speak to me. What came out of the conversation was that the green face was angry at Claire and didn't want her to dance.

To hold the energy at this point, it was not necessary for me to go into "anger" but rather to feel my corresponding "force." When I asked why he didn't want Claire to dance, he made a jump in time, and we were back in medieval times. Claire, now in a deep trance state, experienced what seemed to be several jolts of energy shooting through her body. She could still talk, and the "green monster" described the images he saw. He saw Claire as a woman who lived in the woods and worked with herbs. She enjoyed dancing and singing in nature, celebrating in this way, the deep sense of harmony and connection that she felt.

In between jolts of energy, which now went like electric currents through Claire's body, the "monster" told me how this woman was captured by the Inquisition, tortured terribly, and burned at the stake. As Claire went through this, I was empathetic with her, supporting her in this way. After the green face told me this story, Claire went through strong emotional release for about ten minutes.

During this release, I experienced a shift in energy. Somehow, the green face had changed; the energy felt softer. We spent about fifteen minutes in this new space, just being with the energy; it now felt harmonious, and soft waves of energy seemed to move through her. When I asked her whether she had an image that corresponded to this energy state, her voice was soft and deep, and she described herself as a young woman dressed in white. I experienced a very light and warm feeling in my chest and my heart chakra.

I then asked her how she experienced her chest. It felt warm and light. I asked whether she would like to dance from that space. She rose from the chair and began to move slowly with grace and fluidity through the studio where we were working. The green monster had transformed. Claire now carried the etheric energy of a high priestess archetype. She danced for about fifteen minutes, and then we ended the session. After this session her nightmare did not recur, and she made a major breakthrough as a performer.

In summary, the transformation described here is due to the energetic principles of Voice Dialogue. I went with the "green monster" not because I wanted to change it but simply to get to know it. When one goes deeper into the experience of the energy patterns, remarkable things happen that cannot be predicted or previewed. The interaction of totally going into the experience of energy, through the agency of an energetically attuned facilitator, while the Awareness level is witnessing, is what brings about these transformations.

5

TRANSFORMATION

In this chapter, attention will be paid to the direction the transformational process takes as a result of energetically based Voice Dialogue work over a longer period of time. The conclusions are based on my personal experiences, on my observations, and on reports by others.

INCREASE IN VITALITY

Once the Primary Selves trust the work and begin to relax, the transformation takes place on the three levels of the consciousness process: Awareness, Experience of Energy patterns, and the Ego.

In the dialogue process, we learn to separate our energy patterns from the Ego and to experience them more fully. As a result of this process, the energy patterns become more pronounced and the energy flow in our whole system becomes more dynamic, and as a result a new balance in the personality is created. Blocks in the energy flow caused by the holding down of disowned energy patterns by the Primary Selves will usually disappear in time.

In a typical block, for example, the Primary Selves might be holding down our vulnerability to avoid re-experiencing painful experiences we had as a Child. At the beginning of the work, there is no awareness of this disposition, for the Ego is still identified with the Primary Selves, and the vulnerability is a disowned self. The natural archetypal energy flow between vulnerability and power is blocked.

As soon as the energy moves from the power side to vulnerability and reaches the area where old pain is reactivated, the Primary Selves automatically take over and the energy races back to the power side. This cycle happens, without any awareness, over and over again. It happens not only because of the intensity of the pain but also as a result of past conditioning.

However, as the Awareness comes into operation through the work, the Ego will disidentify from the Primary Selves; the Primary Selves will take a closer look at the situation *now* and will be likely to relax a bit in time. The subject will then be able, in the session, to experience the vulnerability in a safe way. In short, the maneuver the Primary Selves had to make in the past in order to protect the vulnerability is usually required no longer.

The movement toward the vulnerable side can sometimes be painful at first, bringing up sadness and tears, but it is usually not unbearable. The interaction of the subject's awareness and the experiencing of the energy pattern activates the healing process, and the energy pattern will naturally transform to its pure state, from a hurt Child to a simply vulnerable Child. The developing Aware Ego will begin to take care of the vulnerability and hold the tension of the opposites.

The flow in the subject's energy system will increase and flow more harmoniously, enabling him to experience his energy patterns more fully. The subject will gain both the energy that the Primary Selves used to hold down the vulnerability, and the energy of the vulnerability itself.

The same transformation process occurs in the reowning of any disowned self, be it vulnerability, the natural instincts, playfulness or rationality. It brings more vitality to our lives.

Towards the Archetypes

In looking at the qualities and contents of our many different parts, it is necessary to understand that we all carry within us, in the psyche and the unconscious, the inherent potential energies of all possible parts, either as dominant, disowned, or undeveloped parts. The source of each respective energy we call an Archetype. This word was used primarily by Carl Gustav Jung, who defined it as an irrepresentable unconscious, pre-existent form that seems to be part of the psyche and can therefore manifest itself spontaneously anywhere, at any time. Because of its instinctual nature, the archetype underlies the feeling-toned complexes and shares their autonomy. (Jung, 1961, p. 392)

So, according to Jung, an archetype originates in the collective unconscious, which is common to everyone, and everyone carries all the archetypes. These archetypes operate in us as predispositions or tendencies to respond to events in a specific manner. Examples of different archetypes are the Mother archetype, the Father archetype, the Hero, the Rational (ordered) archetype, the Irrational (imaginative) archetype, the Daemonic (which carries our negative responses and energies), the Knower, the Cowboy, the Seductress, and the archetypal patterns of the Son and Daughter, to name a few. All of them describe tendencies that exist within all people as ways of being and of responding.

The matter can also be approached from the perspective of Greek mythology. Each of the Gods and Goddesses is a symbolic representation of a different potential way of using energy, i.e., a different archetype. One example is the god Apollo, the god of knowledge, order and the intellect. Opposite him sits the god of release, experience and ecstasy, Dionysius. Each mythological figure carries certain clearly defined characteristics, and, in general, each of us tends to "serve" certain gods in particular, in our thought processes and in how we express ourselves in the world.

It is important to note, however, that each archetype can have different sides to it. The gods can be angry, sad, happy, kind, vengeful, giving, vulnerable, powerful, etc. Also, for every archetype, there is another archetype that carries the opposing tendency, as exemplified by the polarity of Apollo and Dionysius, i.e., rational versus ecstatic.

Jung refers to archetypes as underlying the complexes, and also refers to an archetype as being the "core" of a complex.

What I have experienced myself and observed in others, is that when the Primary Selves begin to trust the work more, experiences of archetypal energies occur more often both in Voice Dialogue sessions and in life. These experiences can be very powerful, both for the subject and for the facilitator. When such an energy pattern emerges in a session, the conversation might go like this:

Facilitator:	Hello, can you tell us who you are?
Voice:	I am an old man. I have a long, white beard. I am sitting under an old oak tree.
Facilitator:	How long have you been there?
Voice:	I have been here forever. I watch the ages go by. I look at the eternal flow of life and death.
Facilitator:	Does (name of subject) know that you are there?
Voice:	He doesn't know me yet, but I have always been with him.

As the facilitator continues to explore this archetypal energy pattern, he may ask whether it has advice for the subject. He may also choose to explore the often rich imagery that accompanies such voices. At that point, the facilitator may ask the subject to close his eyes to allow the images to emerge. The energy pattern may find itself in a mythological landscape or in between the stars.

In encountering an archetype, the energetic experience is usually much stronger than it is in encountering a subpersonality. The energy fields expand, and powerful energy may channel through the subject. It may be an experience of intense peace, as with the wise old man, or divine sensuality when one meets Aphrodite, goddess of love.

It is this strong energetic quality that alerts the facilitator that he may have come across an archetype.

Sometimes we encounter archetypes directly when we work with dreams. One of my first and most powerful experiences in working with archetypes was in facilitating a woman named Sue. This encounter took place in a house somewhere in the woods of northern California, and I, least of all, expected what happened. Sue told me that she had dreamed of a huge deer, who was standing in a stream, scraping his hooves and looking at her impatiently and angrily. In the session I asked Sue whether she could go back to the dream image. After she had done so, I asked whether she could move to a different place so that I could talk to the deer. She moved to a different place and then began to breathe very slowly and deeply. The energy that started to release was incredibly strong. To my vision, the whole room became pitch black, and the energy almost pushed me out of my chair. When the deer started to speak, his voice was about two octaves lower than Sue's normal speaking voice.

The deer spoke slowly and heavily, radiating power. He said he was angry at Sue for not allowing him to come out and for not listening to him. He pointed out a particular spot in the woods where he would like to be, and required of her to go there so that he could come out. He also said that she could greatly benefit from his strength. Although I had done quite a lot of work with my own instinctual energies, I could barely hold this energy, and I told the deer that I was very impressed with his power.

The deer then looked right through me, and, when he spoke, my ears rang. He said that he saw a tiger in my throat that I should get to know. "You are afraid of the tiger, but it will be your ally." I knew at that moment that the deer was right.

At this point the deer, was really facilitating me. He inducted me more deeply into his powerful instinctual energy, which energized my whole body. At some point, the deer said that he didn't want to stay there; if Sue wanted to meet him, she should go to the place he had pointed out.

We went back to the Ego Space and after a short discussion decided to see which energy pattern was on the other side. When Sue had moved to the new place, another very strong energy pattern started to manifest. This time I perceived a soft, golden light coloring the room. The energy pattern that manifested described itself as a Bodhisattva. It was on earth to guide people towards the light. This too was an amazingly strong energetic experience, and it completely opened my heart chakra. As I later reflected on the session, I realized the profound working of the Yin-Yang principle in the session: from the most powerful nature force to the divine light.

In the years that I have worked with this process, I have encountered many archetypal energy patterns. They may call themselves Aphrodite, Ares, Apollo, they may be animals such as in the aforementioned dream, they may be earth mothers, angels, or nature spirits. What makes them archetypes is the transpersonal nature of their energy.

As people become more familiar with subpersonalities, a deepening takes place in working with them, and by going deeper into the experience of the subpersonalities the archetypal quality of the energy patterns is likely to manifest. A transformation takes place on the level of the energy patterns, from the experience of personally conditioned parts toward the experience of the "core" of the energy patterns, the archetypes. For example, the energy pattern that first described itself as the assertive part of the subject may at some point manifest itself as a full-blown archetypal warrior. The energy pattern that first described itself as the feeling side of the subject may later appear as Aphrodite, goddess of love. Even the Primary Selves may transform in time and radiate the transpersonal vibration of Saturn, Lord of Time and Structure.

This transformation on the level of the energetic experiences does not mean that the subject becomes totally transpersonal and loses the experience of the more personally conditioned parts. Rather, he gets access to the universal quality of their energy. As a result of getting access to the archetypal core of his energy patterns, the dynamics of his energy flow will change. Eventually, a stronger and more vital current will develop between the opposing forces Yin and Yang, revitalizing the entire being of the subject.

The work of the developing Aware Ego becomes more and more interesting, holding the tension of ever-widening opposites, balancing the archetypal forces and experiencing the dynamic energy flow between them. This leads naturally to the embodiment of the aforementioned principles: awareness of body and energy fields, relaxation, centeredness, alignment, and the Yin-Yang principle.

As a result of the deepening of the facilitator's own process, the capacity to facilitate another person's process will increase, as more of the facilitator's energies become available to resonate with the subject's energies in the sessions.

PROTECTION AGAINST INFLATION

Jung introduces us to the phenomenon of inflation, which he defines in the following way:

> *Expansion of the personality beyond its proper limits by identification with the persona or with an archetype. It produces an exaggerated sense of one's self-importance and is usually compensated by feelings of inferiority. (Jung, 1965, p. 396)*

In recent history, we have seen terrible examples of inflation where an archetype takes over the Ego. It is found that, by the ritual of Voice Dialogue, these energy patterns can be explored in a safe way. The method encompasses a strong element of disidentification, crucial to the consciousness process.

By going to the place of Awareness at the end of each session, the subject disidentifies from whatever strong energetic experience he had. The developing Aware Ego will thus be in a position to question and process the information that it gathers in the sessions, and thus does not become a victim to the energy patterns.

TRANSFORMATION AND TRANSMUTATION

Transmutation is defined as the changing of energies from one form to another, as in alchemy. This idea is particularly popular in spiritual disciplines. The concept of transmutation is different from transformation. By transmutation or sublimation people try to change "undesirable" energy patterns into "higher" and more acceptable forms. Assagioli dedicates a chapter to this process in his book *Psychosynthesis*, where he recommends certain exercises to sublimate the sexual impulses.

According to the conceptual framework of Voice Dialogue, on the other hand, the danger with transmutation is that, because it entails an effort of the will, it may lead to the repression of the undesired energy patterns. If the Ego is identified with a cluster of subpersonalities like the "Spiritual Pusher," the Inner Critic, and the Controller, or even with the "Higher Self," the undesired energy patterns will be pushed underground and will lurk in the unconscious waiting for a time to come out and strike back. In this respect, it is important to ask oneself *who* it is in us that wants us to transmute a particular energy pattern.

The use of the idea and practice of transmutation to repress undesired energy patterns will not lead to a balanced unfolding of the totality of our selves. Instead, the unconscious will cook up unpleasant surprises. It simply does not work to try to transmute, for example, the Child in us to a grown-up. According to the consciousness model, the Child is a child and will always be a child. It is an archetypal energy pattern and as such is part of our human condition. What we need is to learn to embrace it; then it may change and transform naturally, perhaps from a hurt Child it may become a happy Child. The transformation that takes place when we learn to embrace it doesn't change the essential nature of the energy pattern. The transformational process is the natural unfolding that takes place on the level and according to the nature of each energy pattern. It is stimulated as a result of the acceptance and nurturing of the energy patterns as they are. If we don't accept our energy patterns as they are, but try instead to force them to change, the natural process of transformation will be blocked. In my experience in this work, I have seen even the most vicious energy patterns transform into their natural archetypal core as a result of accepting them.

TWO CASES

To present an idea of the transformation over a period of time, I will describe two cases of people with whom I have worked.

ANNE

On February 12, 1987, Anne, a 26-year-old woman, came to see me. A few years earlier she had finished her studies to become a schoolteacher, but now she felt quite depressed and didn't feel able to work as a schoolteacher. She regularly experienced sudden fear and panic, sometimes while walking on the street or in a group of people. She was afraid that she would lose control. She was aware of what was going on and to some degree could control her fears. She was also able to reflect on herself. After an initial talk, we decided to work for a while using Voice Dialogue.

In the first session, I worked with her Primary Selves, a very harsh Inner Critic, a Warrior, and a Child that was scared and in great pain.

The Primary Selves were willing to let me talk to other parts of Anne. The next part that came up was the Vulnerable Child, but I was able to catch only a glimpse of it before, almost immediately, the Inner Critic moved in. It really hated the Child and recounted all the times that the Child had made Anne feel embarrassed, until finally she had managed to bury it. These stories had to do with Anne's childhood and her experiences at school. The Critic worked in various ways: she spoke to Anne and also had a variety of ways to let Anne feel physically that she was not O.K. We really "stretched" the Critic until finally Anne's Ego came in and said that this was enough. She was surprised and angry at the control the Inner Critic had.

We then talked to a part that was strong, had self-esteem, and could try to protect the Child from all this Criticism. This part had a Warrior-like instinctual quality. From there, we went to the Child. As she first came out, she could not speak but just curled up in a corner, quite scared. After just being there for a while, we moved back to the Ego. When I reviewed the session, Anne, standing in the place of Awareness, had quite some insights. When we returned to the Ego space, she told me that, in the place of Awareness, she recognized that the energy of the Critic was like her mother, who had completely disowned her vulnerability. Anne realized that the condition the Child was in was due to her own sudden panics.

In the following months, we worked once a week. The process was a continuation of what had happened in the first session. The Inner Critic came out regularly, as did the Warrior and the Child.

As Anne learned to separate more from the Critic, its energy started to change. At some point, it became sad and was afraid that it would have no more place in Anne's life. The Critic didn't think this was fair, as all it had done was to try to protect her. The Warrior grew stronger, which was visible in Anne's body and energy system.

The Child was in great pain when it first came out, but just letting it be in its space had a transforming effect. In fact, the Child gradually felt less scared and also began to speak. As Anne developed more awareness of all these energy patterns, she was able in her daily life to be more with the Child, even if it was in pain. The sessions brought up a lot of insight regarding Anne's painful childhood situation.

Later, an archetypal mother figure came out in one of our sessions and began to take care of the Child.

After a few months of weekly sessions, the Child was no longer scared but just vulnerable and enjoyed being present. The Child was very sensitive and gave her a new connection to nature. The Critic did not disappear but transformed and became a part of the discerning mind. Anne's sudden fears and panics had gradually disappeared.

During the six month period in which we worked, Anne's process was reflected in her dreams.

The Child was a very important theme. In the first dream, Anne found a very sick child in her kitchen; Anne didn't want to take care of the child but also couldn't get rid of her. In later dreams, the child was still ill, but Anne had begun to take care of her. Still later, the child was healthy and they were playing together. In the last dream the child was magical, and showed her how to fly.

From a transformational point of view, several energy patterns transformed: the Critic became milder, the Warrior stronger, the wounds of the Child healed, and even some "new" energies developed. Anne also had more Awareness and was able to make real choices from an Aware Ego.

BOB

On October 10, 1986, Bob, 28 years old, joined one of my ongoing groups in Amsterdam. After studying acupuncture and homeopathy, he had just started to practise. He was also practising meditation. He joined my group for personal growth and to find out whether he could use Voice Dialogue in his beginning practice.

During the course of the work, he recognized that his intense dislike of aggressive and violent people might have to do with a disowned self. He, himself, was very sensitive and kind. I worked with him regularly in the group over a period of five months. The initial reason for him to work on the subject of aggression was the following dream:

"It is nighttime, and I am walking along a highway. On the other side of the road, two men are having an argument. I come closer and watch them argue. I feel very uncomfortable. They are very angry at each other. Then one man picks up a pitchfork and rams it right through the other one's chest. I feel nauseated and wake up sweating."

From this dream, it seemed obvious to me that what needed to be integrated in Bob were his demonic and instinctual energies. When I talked about the dream with him in the Ego place, his Controller was very present, and so was the frightened Child. In this first session, I worked only with the Controller, the Pleaser and the Child, because these energies were not ready to let the aggressive part come in. The Controller and Pleaser were not only afraid to lose control if Bob moved to the aggressive part, but also found the part utterly despicable. The Controller worked in collaboration with the Pleaser, whose job it is to make sure that people like Bob. In early childhood, Bob had learned this way to take care of his vulnerability, and it was still in operation. The Child was quite scared and needed to be taken care of.

In the next session, two weeks later, I worked again with the Controller and the Child. We also looked for a part of Bob that could help him take better care of the Child. A beautiful Mother energy emerged and was very sensitive to the needs of this inner Child.

When Bob got more awareness of these parts, disidentified from the Controller and Pleaser and learned to take better care of his inner Child, he was ready for the next step. Meanwhile, he regularly had dreams to do with the theme of the demonic and instinctual energies. One of the dreams was as follows:

"I live in a house where several people live. Somebody has been murdered and cut up into little pieces. The pieces are put in a plastic garbage bag. The bag with the chopped-up body is put in my room. I feel terribly worried about this and in a strange way also guilty, as if I have been involved in the killing too, but I don't know how. I throw the bag out of the window, which luckily nobody notices. I wake up feeling sick and guilty."

In the next session, I talked to the Controller again, and the Controller was then willing to let me talk to a part of Bob that was selfish and not nice. I explored the Selfish Voice, had him freely express his feelings about people Bob knows, and found out that this voice likes different clothes, likes to have a fast car and a lot of money. We had made our entry into the realm of the instinctual.

In later sessions, we explored various other aspects of this realm, such as the sexual part and the part that would like to steal. In the process, I regularly checked in with the Primary Selves. In each session we ventured a little further, until after a few months, we also explored the demonic. In Bob's case, we worked with sadistic sexual fantasies.

Meanwhile, Bob continued having dreams of violence. I want to describe here the last dream of the series, because it constellated a true transformation of energies that were visible in Bob's entire being:

"I am walking in the center of Amsterdam. There is a lot of commotion and tension on the streets; people are walking nervously around, hurrying home. I ask a friend why everyone is so tense. She says that there is a killer loose, but nobody knows where he is or when he is going to strike again. The police are checking everyone. My friend doesn't like it. I quite understand the police. I take a tram and someone opens beer bottles, the beer spraying all around. I don't understand why, as I feel nervous with this killer around.

"Suddenly, I am somewhere else. I am walking on a hill with two people, a boy and a girl. As we walk together up the hill, I suddenly become very suspicious. The thought comes up that one of them may be the killer.

"Then they disappear and I walk alone over a meadow. As I walk for a while, suddenly, the thought strikes me that perhaps *I* am the killer. As this realization comes, I suddenly feel a tremendous energy rising from my guts that totally possesses me. My face contorts, my body changes, I grow claws, I change into a werewolf. I am the killer, and I need to kill somebody. As I proceed like this, I see a man sleeping in the grass. As I walk towards him, I raise my right claw. I strike downward with tremendous force. As soon as I hit his body, the whole scene changes. The man and I dissolve into pure energy, creating a powerful vibrating sound. This ball of sound that we become travels through space, giving me an intense feeling of power and luminosity.

"I wake up feeling totally energized."

This dream marked the end of a cycle. Bob looked like a new person, he radiated a different energy, and he became very successful in his work. As a facilitator, I simply followed Bob's energies, resonated with them, and induced him every time a little deeper and further into them. Via the Primary Selves, the Pleaser, the Child, and the Mother, we eventually arrived at the instinctual. It is a very organic process. Following the principles described earlier in the facilitation, such a process goes beyond therapy and is truly a journey of discovery. In this case, it was a transformation of Demonic energies, which had previously been disowned, back to their root, pure instinctual power.

EXPERIMENTS IN DAILY LIFE

In the course of the work, as the Ego becomes more and more aware, it processes the information received from the awareness level and the experiences of the different energy patterns. It learns to hold the tension of opposites and does not need to act automatically under the whim of a manifesting energy pattern.

On the other hand, in the daily life, a person with a developed Aware Ego may choose, after careful consideration, to drop into an energy pattern in order to explore it fully.

To clarify this point, I will use an experience of my own, described in my journal, dated September 9, 1984:

"When I came back to Amsterdam in 1984 after studying with Hal Stone for nine months in Los Angeles, things did not work out for me as I had expected. I was trying to organize work as a trainer, but not enough people signed up for the workshops I had organized. I had the feeling that I didn't receive the help I needed from other people. I also found it hard to adjust to living in Amsterdam again.

"After some introspection, I became aware of the fact that I felt victimized. I was also aware that my Primary Self did not like me to become a victim and was trying to repress this energy pattern by trying to hold it down.

"I became aware of these opposite energies at work in me, but the dynamics of Primary Selves and Victim did not change, nor did the actual work situation. I felt stuck, and one morning I made the following choice: I said, 'O.K., if there is this Victim in me, I'd better become this Victim totally. Let's see what happens.'

"I asked the Primary Self for his permission, which he gave because he said he was getting tired, and I then allowed myself to be fully pulled by the gravity of the Victim. I didn't need to drop consciously: just letting go of the Controller did the job. I found that allowing the Victim to be totally present was already of some relief, for I didn't have to fight it any more. I now started to experience the world completely from the perspective of the Victim.

"That morning I went out to ride on my bike to a nice village by a river, about ten miles from Amsterdam. The first thing that went wrong was that I got lost on my way out of Amsterdam. Instead of enjoying a nice ride along the river, I ended up riding in an industrial area with trucks driving on and off. Then I followed a road sign in the direction of the village, only to find myself, after a long time, between huge apartment buildings. Eventually, I arrived at the village. On my way back to Amsterdam I had a flat tire, which I had to repair at the side of the road. I finally arrived back in Amsterdam in the middle of the rush hour. In the evening at home, it was not hard to indulge fully in being the Victim, feeling pity for myself and everything that went wrong in my life. Finally, I reached the depths of the energy pattern. The feeling then miraculously disappeared, and I no longer felt a victim.

"I had become so familiar with the Victim that now, in a strange way, I missed my relationship to it."

By consciously choosing to go fully into the experience of the energy pattern, the energy pattern had somehow transformed, and the dynamic energy flow between power and vulnerability had been restored. After the experience, my Primary Selves didn't need to hold the Victim down any more; there was no more fear and waste of energy.

I also realized that I had to take better care of my inner Child, I felt a lot more strength to act in the world, and within a relatively short time, my work started to flourish.

What the example shows is that under certain conditions one can be one's own facilitator. The Aware Ego can choose to experiment with the energy patterns in daily life. The same energetic principles then come into operation as in the Voice Dialogue sessions.

Depending on the nature of the energy patterns at work, experiments like this one can vary from painful, when we experience a hurt Child, to very exciting, as in the case of the Warrior. However, no energetic state is permanent, and at some point the energy will shift.

ARTISTS OF LIFE

Choices made from an Aware Ego level to honor our selves can allow us, in the case of our Inner Child, to spend an afternoon at the sea, to buy ice cream, or to go to the cinema. In order to allow our more extraverted selves to be there, we may buy clothes that they like and take them out to a party.

When we reach the state of making such choices, life becomes a stage and we become artists of life. The options we have available are determined by the course of our own individual process and the energy patterns that manifest in that course. We learn to be more in tune with what is going on inside us and more aware of the energy patterns outside us, in the world, that correspond to these inner states. From an Aware Ego level we can now make choices concerning our actions in the world in order to "feed" certain parts of ourselves.

Charles, after working in my groups for a year, came to the conclusion that his earlier choice to become a psychotherapist had not been made from an Aware Ego. He took care of other people because he could not take care of his own vulnerable Child. After he learned how to take care of it, his next important insight was that he had completely disowned his power side. The power side came out in sessions many times, but it wanted more expression than it could get, at that point, either in the sessions or in his life. After examining the issue from different perspectives in several sessions, Charles decided to give up his work as a psychotherapist and to accept a job he had been offered in the Amsterdam stock market. He has been working there quite successfully for a year now.

By experiencing and working with Voice Dialogue, people can become aware and learn to embody basic principles of transformation.

The profound energetic experiences and the insights people get in the sessions contribute to the larger process of transformation throughout their lives. This larger evolutionary process of transformation, continually changing and fluctuating, takes place over time on many levels of consciousness. It cannot be programmed, there will always be new energy patterns that manifest in the course of the journey, coming either from the inside, as through a dream, or from the outside, through new people that we meet, as well as through the unexpected challenges that the life process provides.

By understanding that *energy follows thought* and through the embodiment of the energetic principles of resonance, induction, *relaxation, centeredness, alignment* and the *Yin-Yang principle*, we will learn—as in the practice of Tai Chi Ch'uan—to find harmony and balance in the world.

A person with a developing Aware Ego will be in a position of having choice, making choices, and living the grand experiment. He will be able to use various approaches and strategies in its explorations of the inner and outer worlds. These strategies can include different forms of therapy, spiritual practices, travelling to different countries, or choosing different work situations.

He will be able to live life to the fullest, meeting the different gods and goddesses as he reaches the core of each energy pattern in the process of the work. At the same time, he can be utterly amazed at it all.

6

SUMMARY, CONCLUSIONS, & RECOMMENDATIONS FOR FURTHER RESEARCH

In order to set a foundation for the greater development of the energetics aspects of the Stone-Winkelman consciousness model, this thesis has explored both that consciousness model and the basic components of the Voice Dialogue method. In addition, a historical overview has been given of the traditions that contributed to its perspective.

The axioms used in the esoteric healing tradition, which rely upon the language of the aura and the chakras, have been explored as the basic principles of energy work.

The basic principles of T'ai Chi Ch'uan, as described in the T'ai Chi Ch'uan Classics, have been explored and demonstrated. The different phases in a Voice Dialogue session have been described in detail, as have two energetically based sessions, in order to clarify the energetic principles that make the work effective.

It has been observed that these basic Voice Dialogue principles correlate with the axioms of the esoteric healing tradition and with the T'ai Chi Chuan principles.

Furthermore, it has been brought out that the following energetic principles must be embodied for the Voice Dialogue facilitator to do *real* transformational work:

1) awareness of body and energy fields
2) the axiom that energy follows thought
3) resonance
4) induction
5) alert relaxation
6) centeredness
7) alignment
8) the Yin-Yang principle

In the example cases presented, it has been shown and demonstrated that, if the facilitator has good proficiency in the use of energetics, the natural flow of the subject's psychic energy is likely to be restored. Furthermore, energetically based Voice Dialogue work will at the same time help the subject to gain access to the natural, archetypal core of the energy patterns. In this way, the life process of the subject is deepened. Two cases presented illustrate this level of the work.

As a result of working with Voice Dialogue in an energetic way over a longer period of time, people gain a new perspective on their lives. The usual perception of the separation between the inner and outer worlds changes, and the subject is able to experience his own energy patterns more fully and is aware of the energy patterns in the world that resonate with these inner states. He will, therefore, be in a position to participate more fully and at a deeper level of functioning in his individual environment.

Based on the framework of this study, it is hoped that further studies may emerge that focus on the exploration of specific energy patterns, such as vulnerability and the instinctual energies, and their relationships to the body energy fields and the chakra system.

It is hoped that new techniques will emerge that can produce more scientifically based experiments in tracking the movements of the energy fields, and, therefore, lead to a better understanding of the nature of the dynamics of energy patterns in consciousness work.

It must be recognized, also, that this brief exploration of the importance of energetics in consciousness work may be only the beginning of a much larger investigation into the nature of psychological reality based on an energetic perspective. In this perspective, insights from various traditions can be investigated and included in the larger work of Transformational Psychology.

ENERGETIC TRAINING

In addition to the "natural" induction into the energetics of Voice Dialogue through work in the sessions with experienced facilitators, specific training in energetics greatly helps people become more aware of the energetic principles of the method and thus stimulates them to work more energetically. The energetic principles should be introduced fairly early in group work; they give the work a new dimension. The exercises clearly demonstrate and give people the experience of the energetic principles of Voice Dialogue. The effect of the exercises on later sessions is quite evident.

EXERCISES BASED ON T'AI CHI CH'UAN

To introduce awareness of the basic principles for the facilitation, I use some preliminary exercises from T'ai Chi that demonstrate the T'ai Chi principles. These principles are not only a metaphor for the principles of the facilitation, but the practice of T'ai Chi also helps to embody them. In fact, a good many people in the Netherlands who were introduced to these principles through Voice Dialogue energetic training have started to take T'ai Chi lessons and are now avid practitioners.

EXERCISE 1: STANDING

Stands with the feet placed parallel to each other at shoulder width and with the knees slightly bent. In this posture, try to relax. Imagine a line from the top of your head running downward through your body into the ground. Standing in this way, simply to let go of the tensions in your body by imagining them dropping down the imaginary line into the earth. If the exercise is done correctly, the breathing will become calm, the abdomen will relax, you will get a sense of *center* in the waist, and the mind will relax.

This preliminary exercise focuses on principles of relaxation, alignment and centering. The teacher will come by and help to correct the posture if a person stands too much forward or backward. The teacher can also help people become aware of the holding of unnecessary tension in the various parts of the body, e.g., the shoulders. By consciously going to the tense part of the body with the mind, you can let go of the tension, visualizing it flowing downward along the line into the earth.

EXERCISE 2: WALKING

Starting from the standing position, holding the knees slightly bent and the spine straight, slowly start to shift the weight to one leg (the "full" leg) until you feel no weight in the other (the "empty" leg). Once the weight is fully on one leg, shift the weight back to the other leg. In continuing to shift the weight from one leg to the other, try to find a natural rhythm, moving like the pendulum of a clock.

Awareness should be totally in the movement, focusing on what happens to the body as a result of this rhythmic shifting. If you can relax and be aligned while doing it, you will begin to feel a flow of energy, originating in the legs. The more you can relax and let the weight sink totally into each alternate leg, the stronger the flow will be. At some point, the movement will feel as if it is happening totally by itself. Now, you can start to lift the "empty" leg and make a step, then sink the weight into the same leg so that it is now "full," and make another step with the other leg, moving in the rhythm that you have found.

Walk in this way, moving from the waist, following this natural rhythm. The fluctuation of "full" and "empty" will activate the energy flow in the entire body.

This exercise makes people aware of what is called the Yin-Yang principle in T'ai Chi. If you go fully into one polarity, in this case by shifting the weight to one leg, the polarity between the Yin and Yang increases, and the energy at some point has to move back to the other polarity. In T'ai Chi, this walking exercise is the basis of all the other movements and forms that follow. In Voice Dialogue, as has been explained, the Yin-Yang principle really is the key to the work, and a proper understanding and embodiment of this principle by the practitioner gives the work its transformative nature.

EXERCISE 3: YIELDING

The next exercise is done in pairs. Two people, A and B, stand facing each other. Person A stands, relaxed and firm, with eyes closed. Person B now pushes A gently on different parts of the body. Person A lets himself be pushed without losing balance. If Person A is relaxed and centered, he will be able to yield to the pushing of Person B. In the beginning, Person B pushes lightly. If A is able to yield at this stage, B can push a little harder and move a little faster. For A, the exercise is a training in the aforementioned principles—relaxation, alignment, centeredness, Yin-Yang principle. It is a training in moving with energies without letting these energies put one out of balance. Later, A and B reverse roles and go through the process again.

The same attitude of yielding with energies while holding center is required of the Voice Dialogue facilitator; therefore this exercise is a good metaphor for the Voice Dialogue work. Often, when people do this exercise they are too "hard": they resist the pushes with force instead of yelding to the incoming energy, and, if the opponent is stronger, they lose their balance. The exercise shows that the principles of T'ai Chi make it possible to move and dance with energies without losing oneself.

EXERCISES BASED ON WORKING WITH BODY-ENERGY FIELDS

Another kind of exercise is used to examine the relationships between subpersonalities and archetypes on the one side and the different chakras on the other side. These exercises are based on the axiom that energy follows thought.

1: EXPLORING THE CHAKRAS

The members of the group sit relaxed, on chairs or the floor, as they prefer. The teacher asks them to bring their attention to various parts of the body and to the different chakras systematically, one by one. Start with the first chakra and gradually proceed till the seventh. The teacher describes the area where the chakra is situated and ask them to focus on it. Each person brings attention to the area and just notices what comes up—images, feelings, sensations, thoughts, whatever. The teacher then asks the group to focus on whatever came up with the chakra, let it grow, and see if a "character" or subpersonality emerges that corresponds to these perceptions. The participants then share their experiences, either in pairs or in the group as a whole.

The exercise is done with all the major chakras along the spine. It is not necessary before the exercise to go into the meaning and functions attributed to the different chakras. It is a simple exercise of awareness, that brings up a lot of experiences; people see, feel, smell things; they discover which areas feel comfortable and which areas do not. (Incidentally, the many reports of experiences of the different chakras of people who knew nothing about chakras seem to confirm that the ideas and functions attributed to the chakras by the esoteric traditions are right.) After they have noted what subpersonality comes up with each chakra, people can explore them in more detail later in a Voice Dialogue session.

In the same manner as with the chakras, one can focus on parts of the body to see what emerges. This process can be particularly powerful if the focus is on a painful spot or area in the body. Quite unexpected images and "characters" can come up. From a painful spot in the neck, the Inner Critic may emerge; by focusing on a sore spot in the stomach, one may get in touch with anger that needs to be released. This exercise also makes it clear how Voice Dialogue can be incorporated in massage and body work.

2) SHIELDING AND EXPANDING ENERGY

The next series of exercises is done in pairs. In this one, two people sit facing each other, about two feet apart, with their eyes closed. Each person imagines an impenetrable shield all around his own body that can protect against any outside influences. The actual image that serves to produce protection varies from person to person. Some imagine a glass or crystal ball, some an iron gate, and the Kahunas in Hawaii use the image of a crystal wall covered with earth on which grass grows. A woman in one of my groups imagined a thick white fur coat that covered her all over. Both people in the pair now experience their own energy in this state for a little while. Then the teacher suggests that they gradually take their shields away, imagine their energy fields expanding, and see how this feels and what happens in their experience of energy. As the energy expands, each will feel the energy of the other person. Then they can withdraw their energy again and expand a few times to feel the difference. Afterward, some time should be allowed for the partners to share their experiences.

This simple exercise usually brings up a lot. People experience that indeed energy follows thought, and by opening up energetically, their energy starts to resonate with the energy of their partners.

3) SENDING AND RECEIVING ENERGY

In this exercise, done in pairs, Person A first shields while Person B consciously expands and sends energy to try to reach A. Person A then gradually takes away the shield to allow B in; A and B pay close attention to what happens in their bodies and energy fields while this takes place. This also can be done a few times, one sending and the other opening and closing. Then the roles are reversed and the exercise repeated.

Here again time should be allowed to share the experience, for this exercise can bring up some emotions having to do with being rejected when the other one closes off energetically. Some people have difficulty closing off energetically, and others find it difficult to send.

There are variations on this exercise. People can send energy from different chakras and to different areas of the partner. The exercise clearly demonstrates the axiom that energy follows thought, and it trains people in using their ability to direct it.

4) SUBPERSONALITIES AND ENERGY FIELDS

Another set of exercises trains people to consciously "drop into" (or "sink into") the energy of the subpersonalities and to be aware of changes in another person's energy field.

Two people sit facing each other, eyes closed. Person A is neutral and receptive. Person B will be going to drop into different subpersonalities which the teacher specifies. An energy pattern to start with is the Primary Selves. B allows this energy pattern to manifest fully in the body and energy system. B will now be radiating this energy. Person A will now be receiving it and will try to be aware of how it affects his energy system. The teacher then suggests that Person B let go of the Primary Selves and invite some other energy to come in, e.g., the playful Child. Person B lets this energy manifest fully in his body, maybe sits differently and just feels it. Person A, meanwhile, is aware of possible changes that he may experience while he feels Person B's energy. Different parts of A's energy field and body will start to resonate with B's playful child energy.

The same thing can be done with other energy patterns; one may evoke for example, the instinctual parts or the emotional ones. At the end, A and B share their experiences and reverse their roles.

After this exercise, a variation is possible in which Person B drops into an energy pattern and Person A simply by feeling its energy, guesses what kind of subpersonality it is. This can be done with different subpersonalities.

After people have done the preliminary exercises, it is amazing how fast they learn to guess correctly.

For the sender, this exercise extends the ability to evoke and drop into subpersonalities at will, and, for the receiver, it increases the receptivity and capacity to resonate with different energy patterns; both skills are important for Voice Dialogue facilitators. Here again, the principle involved is that energy follows thought.

There are many variations possible on the exercises described. One can, for example, have the receiver tune into the energy pattern that is received, drop into that part, and send the same energy back.

DEFINITION OF TERMS

Archetype
One of many patterns of life that are universally valid; represented in myth, in story form. Primordial possibility for action, or psychic predisposition for the shaping of response.

Aura or Energy Field
W.E. Butler writes: "A subtle invisible essence or fluid that emanates from human or animal bodies, and even from things; a psychic electro-vital, electro-mental effluvium, partaking of both mind and body."

Awareness
The capacity of witnessing life in all its aspects without evaluating or judging the energy patterns being witnessed and without having the need to control the outcome of an event.

Chakras
Distribution centers through which the vital energy drawn from the sun and the earth by the etheric body is passed into the physical body. To a clairvoyant these centers look like whirlpools or trumpet-shaped vortices of energy.

Chi
Vital energy or life force.

Consciousness
Both the awareness and the experience of energy patterns.

Disowned Selves
Those selves or energy patterns that have been partially or totally excluded from one's life.

Ego and Aware Ego

The ego is the executive function of the psyche, or the choice-maker. It receives its information both from the Awareness level and from the experience of the different energy patterns. As one moves forward in the consciousness process, the ego becomes a more Aware Ego. As a more Aware Ego, it is in a better position to make real choices.

Energetics

The science that deals with the laws of energy and its transformations, when applied psychologically, it relates to the study of energy systems within the personality construct.

Energy

Internal or inherent power; the power of operating, whether exercised or not.

Energy Pattern

The homogeneous structure on which everything else is based.

Induction

Beyond the dictionary meaning, "the process by which a body having electric or magnetic properties produces magnetism, an electric charge or an electromotive force in a neighboring body, without contact," this term is used in a psychological sense, that is, the process of an individual's holding an awareness or maintaining a presence in such a manner that it may be transmitted to another.

Primary Selves

The selves or energy patterns with which we have identified ourselves in order to survive psychologically.

Resonance

In addition to the dictionary definition, "reinforcement and prolongation of a sound by reflection or by vibration of other bodies", the use of this word also includes: two or more individual's establishing a sense of rapport and alignment of energies.

Subpersonalities

A variety of little networks of behaviors, seen as specific personality parts that are real, self-governing, and independent within the totality of the larger construct of personality.

T'ai Chi Ch'uan

A Chinese martial art based on the principles of Taoism. Literally, the supreme, ultimate art of boxing. T'ai Chi Ch'uan is a method by which external affairs are regulated (self-defense) while the Chi (vital energy) is cultivated.

Transformation

A change that results in a nonsuperficial alteration in either a person, a group or a culture. Such a change is neither unusual nor unnatural but is characteristic of the essential nature of reality. Furthermore, this alteration is not value-free but is in a direction that enhances the organism and supports its participation in a wider context and greater wholeness of life.

To Align

To consciously connect with the spheres of heaven and earth in order to establish a balanced position that will enable one to let go of superfluous energy into the earth and take in energy from both heaven and earth.

To Drop Into

The internal action of the Voice Dialogue facilitator to move into one of his own energy patterns in order to bring it forward physically and energetically. This action requires a conscious intention and uses the inherent "gravity" of the energy patterns. This technique is used to enable induction.

Yin-Yang Principle

The principle that energy always flows between the opposite polarities of the Yin (negative) and Yang (positive). When the energy has fully flown to one side of the polarity, it will naturally shift back to the other side of the polarity.

BIBLIOGRAPHY

Assagioli, R. (1965). *Psychosynthesis.*
New York: Viking Press.

Brandon, N. (1972). *The Disowned Self.*
New York: Nash Publishing Co.

Burr, H.S. (1972). *Blueprint for Immortality.*
London: Spearman.

Butler, W.E. (1971). *How to Read the Aura.*
London: Aquarian Press.

Chen Wei-ming. *Commentary on Yang Cheng-fu's Ten Important Points.*
In Lo et al. (1979), p. 87.

De Miranda, Y. (1983). *An aerial view of archetypes and subpersonalities with an inquiry into psycho-spiritual androgyny.*
Unpublished doctoral dissertation, International College, Los Angeles.

Fordham, F. (1953). *An Introduction to Jung's Psychology.*
Hammondsworth, Middlesex: Penguin Books, Ltd.

Hamilton, E. (1940). *Mythology.*
New York: Mentor.

Joy, W.B. (1979). *Joy's Way: A Map for the Transformational Journey.*
Los Angeles: J. P. Tarcher.

Jung, C.G. (1933). *Modern Man in Search of a Soul.*
New York: Harcourt, Brace, Jovanovich.

Jung, C.G.(1961). *Memories, Dreams, Reflections.*
New York: Vintage Books.

Koolbergen, J. (1973). *Growth Therapy: Model and Exercises.*
Unpublished doctoral dissertation, University of Amsterdam, The Netherlands.

Krippner, S., & Rubin, D. (1975). *The Energies of Consciousness.*
New York: Interface Books.

Krishnamurti, J. (1954). The first and last freedom. Wheaton, IL:
The Philosophical Publishing House.

Krishnamurti, J. (1968). *The Awakening of Intelligence.*
New York: Harper & Row.

Krishnamurti, J. (1972). Talk at Stanford University, *You Are the World.*
New York: Harper & Row, p. 150.

Kushi, M. (1973). *Acupuncture, Ancient and Future Worlds.*
Boston: East West Foundation.

Lo, B.P.J., Inn, M., Amacker, R., & Foe, S. (Trans. & Eds.). (1979).
The Essence of Tai Chi Ch'uan.
Richmond, CA.: North Atlantic Books.

Monte, C. E. (1980). *Beneath the Mask.*
New York: Holt, Rinehart & Winston.

Nicoll, M. (1952). *Psychological Commentaries on the Teachings of Gurdjieff and Ouspensky* (Vol 1).
London: Vincent Stuart.

Nifenger, L. A. (1985). *The Emerging Role of the Transformational Psychologist in our Society.*
Unpublished master's thesis, International College, Los Angeles.

Ornstein, R. E. (1972). *The Psychology of Consciousness.*
San Francisco: Freeman & Co.

Ostrander, S., & Schroeder, L. (1971). *Psychic Discoveries Behind the Iron Curtain.*
New York: Bantam Books.

Russell, E. (1972). *Plan van Bestemming.*
Kluwer: Deventer.

Stone, H. (1985). *Embracing Heaven and Earth.*
Marina del Rey, CA.: Devorss & Co.

Stone, H., & Winkelman, S. (1985). *Embracing Our Selves.*
Marina del Rey, CA, Devorss & Company.

Tart, C. (1974). *Transpersonal Psychologies.*
New York: Harper & Row.

Unknown author. Song of the thirteen postures.
In Lo et al. (1979), p. 64.

Wang Tsung-yueh. T'ai Chi Ch'uan lun.
In Lo et al. (1979), p. 38.

Wu Yu-hsiang. Expositions of insights into the practice of the thirteen postures.
In Lo et al. (1979), p. 43.

About the Author

Robert Stamboliev studied at the University of Utrecht and with Dr. Hal Stone at William Lyon University in San Diego where he received an M.A. degree in Transformational Psychology.

In 1984, he introduced Voice Dialogue in the Netherlands and Western Europe. He is the Director of the Institute for Transformational Psychology (ITP) in Amsterdam. For information, call or write:

I.T.P.
Instituut voor Transformatie Psychologie
Pieter de Hoochstraat 18
P.O. Box 74038
1070 BA Amsterdam
Telephone: 31-20-6762111 • Fax: 31-20-6752926

Hal Stone, PhD and Sidra Stone, PhD
DELOS, Inc.
P.O. Box 604
Albion, California 95410
Telephone: 818/763-8028 • Fax: 818/763-8086

Delos, Inc. is the name of the organization that encompasses the training, publishing and consultation activities of Drs. Hal and Sidra Stone, the founders of Voice Dialogue. For information regarding any of these programs or publications, please write to the above address.

Books Published:

>Embracing Heaven and Earth, DeVorss and Co., 1984
>Embracing Our Selves, New World Library, 1985, 1989
>Embracing Each Other, New World Library, 1991
>Meet Your Inner Critic (tentative title), forthcoming 1993

Tapes Published:

The Mendocino Series includes 12 audio cassette tapes:
Meeting Your Selves—The Dance of the Selves in Relationship—The Child Within—Meet Your Inner Critic (1 & 2)—Meet Your Pusher—Understanding Relationships—Integrating the Daemonic—Decoding Your Dreams—The Daemonic in Dreams—Introducing Voice Dialogue—Voice Dialogue Demonstrations

Training Activities:

The Drs. Stone conduct various training activities at their home in Northern California, as well as in various teaching centers in the U.S. and abroad. These vary in length between one day and two weeks.

Individual and Couples Consultation:

An intensive program of individual work is available at their home in Northern California. Both individuals and couples come for periods of time to work intensively on their relationship as a couple or on their personal process as an individual.

LifeRhythm Publications

John C. Pierrakos M.D CORE ENERGETICS
Developing the Capacity to Love and Heal
With 16 pages of four-color illustrations of human auras corresponding to their character structure, 300 pages, $18.95
The therapeutic work of John C. Pierrakos M.D. is based on these principles: 1. The person is a psychsomatic unity; 2. The source of healing lies within the self, not with an outside agency, whether a physician, God, or the power of the cosmos; 3. All of existence forms a unity that moves toward creative evolution, both of the whole and of the countless components. Dr. Pierrakos clarifies for us what can be seen of human energy centers (chakras) and the various energy fields (auras). By relating the pulsation frequencies and colors of the fields of human beings, animals, plants and minerals, he defines the stage of health or dysfunction. Through his experience as a practicing psychiatrist, a body-therapist, Dr. Pierrakos has developed a system for evaluating the state of the human organism in terms of illness and health.

Malcolm Brown, Ph.D. THE HEALING TOUCH
An Introduction to Organismic Psychotherapy
320 pages, 38 illustrations, $16.95
A moving and meticulous account of Malcolm Brown's journey from Rogerian-style verbal psychotherapist to gifted body psychotherapist. Influenced by C.G. Jung, Abraham Maslow, Erich Neumann, Carl Rogers, D.H. Lawrence, and Wilhelm Reich, Dr. Brown developed his own art and science of body psychotherapy with the purpose of re-activating the natural mental/ spiritual polarities of the embodied soul and transcendental psyche. Using powerful case histories as examples, Brown describes in theory and practice the development of his work; the techniques to awaken the energy flow and its integration with the main Being centers: Eros, Logos, the Spritual Warrior and the Hara.

B.Baginski and S. Sharamon REIKI; Universal Life Energy
200 pages, illustrations, $12.95
The roots of Reiki reach far back into the ancient origins of natural healing but the method here has been rediscovered in modern times and is now a widely practiced form of folk medicine used by practitioners, therapists and healers. Reiki is described as the energy which forms the basis of all life. With the help of specific methods, anyone can learn to awaken and activate this universal life energy so that healing and harmonizing energy flows through the hands. Reiki is healing energy in the truest sense of the word, leading to greater individual harmony and attunement to the basic forces of the universe. This book features a unique compilation and interpretation, from the author's experience, of over 200 psychosomatic symptoms and diseases

Cousto THE COSMIC OCTAVE Origin of Harmony
128 pages, 45 illustrations, numerous tables, 24 page scientific appendix, $12.95
Cousto demonstrates the direct relationship of astronomical data, such as the frequency of planetary orbits to ancient and modern measuring systems, the human body, music and medicine. Cousto's scientific work is to be seen in the tradition of Johannes Kepler, whose life work *Harmonices Mundi* he has been able to considerably enlarge upon and improve. This book is compelling reading for those who wonder if a universal law of harmony does exist behind the apparent chaos of life. This book is compelling reading for those who wonder if a universal law of harmony does exist behind the apparent chaos of life

Ron Kurtz **BODY CENTERED PSYCHOTHERAPY:**
THE HAKOMI METHOD
The Integrated Use of Mindfulness, Nonviolence and the Body
212 pages, illustrations, $15.95

Some of the origins of Hakomi stem from Buddhism and Taoism, especially concepts like gentleness, compassion, mindfulness, and going with the grain. Other influences come from general systems theory, which incorporates the idea of respect for the wisdom of each individual as a living organic system that spontaneously organizes matter and aenergy and selects from the environment what it needs in a way that maintains its goals, programs and identity. Hakomi is really a synthesis of philosophies, techniques and approaches that has its own unique artistry, form and organic process.

Helmut G. Sieczka **CHAKRA BREATHING**
A Pathway to Energy and Harmony
100 pages Illustrations $10.95   Supplemental Cassette Tape $10.95

A guide to self-healing, this book is meant to help activate and harmonize the energy centers of the subtle body. Through the practice of chakra breathing we can learn to explore and recognize our innate possibilities, uncovering hidden energy potentials. The breath is the bridge between body and soul. In today's world as our lives are determined by stressful careers and peak performance, the silent and meditative moments have become more vital. We can try to remember our true selves more often, so that our natural energy balances can be restored. Chakra-breathing enhances this kind of awareness and transformational work, especially on the emotional and energetic level.

Reinhard Flatischler **THE FORGOTTEN POWER OF RHYTHM**
160 pages, illustrations,$14.95 Supplemental CD $16.95 Cassette $12.95

Rhythm is the central power of our life; it connects us all. There is a powerful source of rhythmic knowledge in every human being, and as we find our way back to this ancient wisdom, we unite with the essence of our life. Reinhard Flatischler presents his revolutionary approach to rhythm in this new book for both the layman and professional musician. TA KE TI NA offers an experience of the interaction of pulse, breath, voice, walking and clapping which awakens our inherent rhythm in the most direct way—through the body. It provides a first hand knowledge of the rhythmic roots of all cultures and a new understanding of the many musical voices of our world.

Fran Brown **LIVING REIKI: TAKATA'S TEACHINGS**
Stories from the Life of Hawayo Takata
100 pages $12.95

In this loving memoir to her teacher, Fran Brown has gathered the colorful stories told by Hawayo Takata during her thirty-five years as the only Reiki Master teaching. The stories create an inspirational panorama of Takata's teachings, filled with the practical and spiritual aspects of a life given to healing.

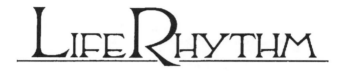

LIFE RHYTHM

Connects you with your Core and entire being—guided by Science, Intuition and Love.

We provide the tools for growth, therapy, holistic health and higher education through publications, seminars and workshops.

If you are interested in our forthcoming projects and want to be on our mailing list, send your address to:

LIFERHYTHM   **P.O. Box 806,**   **Mendocino, CA 95460**
Tel: 707/937-1825   Fax: 707/937-3052